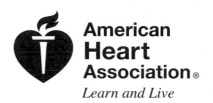

American
Heart
Association®
Learn and Live

Heartsaver®
First Aid CPR AED
STUDENT WORKBOOK

Editors

Louis Gonzales, BS, LP, *Senior Science Editor*

Michael W. Lynch, NREMT-P, *Content Consultant*

Senior Managing Editor

Sue Bork

Special Contributors

Michael A. Buldra

Tony Fernandez, MS, NREMT-P

Susan Fuchs, MD

John Gosford, BS, EMT-P

Theresa Hoadley, RN, PhD, TNS

Scott Larson, EMT

Mary Mast, RN

David Parish, MD, MPH

Adam J. Singer, MD

Mark A. Terry, MPA, NREMT-P

First Aid Subcommittee 2010-2011

Rita Herrington, FNP, *Chair*

Louis Gonzales, BS, LP, *Immediate Past Chair,*
2006-2009

Kostas Alibertis, CCEMT-P

Nate Charlton, MD

Jeffrey D. Ferguson, MD, NREMT-P

Peter Fromm, MPH, RN

Michael Hendricks, EMT

Helen McCracken, RDH, MS

George Murphy, EMT-P

Jeanette Previdi, RN-BC, BSN, MPH

William Smith, MD

Jeff Woodin, NREMT-P

© 2011 American Heart Association
ISBN 978-1-61669-017-5
Printed in the United States of America
First American Heart Association Printing March 2011
10 9 8 7 6 5 4 3

To find out about any updates or corrections to this text, visit **www.heart.org/cpr**, navigate to the page for this course, and click on "Updates."

Contents

CONTENTS

Preface

Welcome to the American Heart Association Heartsaver® First Aid CPR AED Course. This course provides a framework for learning basic skills that may save a life or prevent further injury. As cofounder of the National First Aid Science Advisory board, the AHA is dedicated to decrease death and disability when an emergency happens. The AHA believes that YOU can make a difference. We thank you most sincerely for taking this course.

Our thanks go to the many volunteers and staff who made this course possible. There are not words to express the gratitude felt for their passion, expertise, and countless hours of work.

Rita Herrington, FNP
First Aid Subcommittee Chair

Introduction

What You Will Learn In this course you'll learn:

- First aid basics
- CPR for adults and how to use an AED

You may also learn child and infant CPR. (These two are optional.)

The Learning Process You will learn first aid basics and CPR AED through this Student Workbook and the video for the course.

During the course you'll practice some skills. If you demonstrate that you can do the skills taught in the course, you'll receive a Heartsaver First Aid CPR AED course completion card.

Using This Student Workbook Use this Student Workbook in the following ways:

Before the course:

- Read this Student Workbook.
- Look at the pictures.
- Take notes about your group's policies and procedures. For example, if you work in a facility that has established policies and procedures for emergencies, review these documents and take notes about how this information will apply to you.

During the course:

- Use the Student Workbook to understand the important information and skills taught in the course.

After the course:

- Review the skills frequently.
- Look at the action tables and skills summaries in the Student Workbook. This will help you remember first aid, CPR, and automated external defibrillator (AED) use.

How Often Training Is Needed Review your Student Workbook and Quick Reference Guide often to keep your skills fresh. You need to retake this course every 2 years to get a new course completion card.

If you have a latex allergy, tell your emergency response program supervisor and your instructor before you start the course.

Part 1: First Aid Basics

What You Will Learn   You'll learn the basics of first aid.

Definitions and Key Facts

First aid is the immediate care that you give someone with an illness or injury before someone with more advanced training arrives and takes over.

First aid may help someone recover more completely or more quickly and may mean the difference between life and death.

Most of the time you'll give first aid for minor illnesses or injuries. You may also give first aid for a more serious illness or injury, such as a heart attack or major bleeding.

Topics Covered

- Rescuer Duties
- Victim and Rescuer Safety
- Phoning for Help
- Finding the Problem (*Skill You Will Demonstrate)
- After the Emergency

1. Rescuer Duties

What You Will Learn

In this section we'll cover

- Deciding to Provide First Aid
- Asking to Provide First Aid
- Supplying the First Aid Kit

Deciding to Provide First Aid

Definitions and Key Facts

Some people may be required to perform first aid while working. For example, law enforcement officers, firefighters, flight attendants, lifeguards, and park rangers may have a duty to give first aid when they are working. If they are off-duty, they can choose whether or not to provide first aid.

**Action:
Deciding to
Provide First Aid**

Providing first aid may be part of your job description. If so, you must help while you're working. However, when you're off-duty, you can choose whether or not to provide first aid.

Asking to Give First Aid

**Definitions and
Key Facts**

Before you provide first aid, it's important to ask the ill or injured person if you may help.

Action

Step	Action
1	If the person responds, introduce yourself as a first aid provider before you touch him. Ask if you may help him.
2	If the person agrees, you may give first aid.
3	If the person refuses your help, phone your emergency response number (or 911) and stay with him until someone with more advanced training arrives and takes over.
4	If the person is confused or cannot answer, assume that he would want you to help.

Supplying the First Aid Kit

**Definitions and
Key Facts**

The first aid kit contains supplies that you might need in an emergency.

Not all first aid kits contain the same supplies. Your company will decide what the first aid kit should have in it. At the end of this section, you'll find a sample list of supplies for a first aid kit. This list is from the American National Standards Institute (ANSI), but it is only 1 example of what a company might decide to include in a kit.

**Action:
Supplying the
First Aid Kit**

- Keep the supplies in a sturdy, watertight container that is clearly labeled.
- Know where the first aid kit is.
- Replace what you use so the kit will be ready for the next emergency.
- Check the kit at the beginning of each work period for expired supplies and to make sure it is complete and ready for an emergency.

2. Victim and Rescuer Safety

What You Will Learn In this section we'll cover

- Assessing the Scene
- Washing Hands
- Universal Precautions
- Exposure to Blood
- Taking Off Gloves (*Skill You Will Demonstrate)

Assessing the Scene

Definitions and Key Facts

You may have to give first aid in dangerous places. The ill or injured person may be in a room with poisonous fumes, on a busy street, or in a parking lot.

Before doing anything else, make sure the scene is safe for you and the injured person. Keep looking around to make sure that the scene stays safe. You can't help anyone if you're injured yourself.

Action: Assess the Scene

As you approach the scene, consider the following:

Danger: Look out for danger to you and danger to the injured person. Move the injured person only if she's in danger or if you need to move her to provide first aid or CPR. Move her if you can do so safely.

Help: Look for people who can help you and look for telephones. Have someone phone your emergency response number (or 911). Phone for help yourself if no one else is around.

Who: Who's injured? Figure out how many people are hurt and see if you can tell what happened.

Where: Where are you? Be specific. The emergency response team (or 911) dispatcher will want to know your address, floor, or location in the building or on the property.

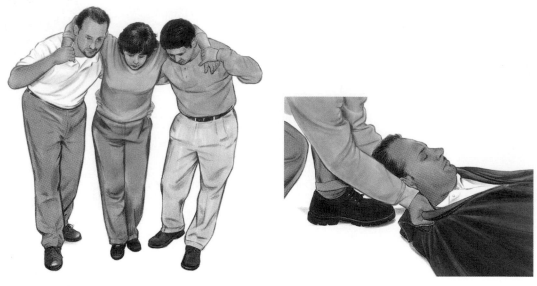

Figure 1. Here are examples of ways to move an ill or injured person.

FYI	When you give first aid, know your limits. Don't become another victim. Sometimes your wish to help can put you in danger. For example, if you are not a good swimmer, be very careful when trying to save someone who's drowning.

Washing Hands

Definitions and Key Facts	Washing your hands well is one of the most important protections you have. Always use soap and water if your hands are visibly dirty and after taking off gloves.

Actions for Washing Hands Well

Step	Action
1	Wet your hands with clean running water (warm if available) and apply soap.
2	Rub hands together and rub all surfaces of hands and fingers for at least 20 seconds.
3	Rinse hands with lots of running water.
4	Dry your hands using a paper towel or air dryer. If possible, use your paper towel to turn off the faucet.

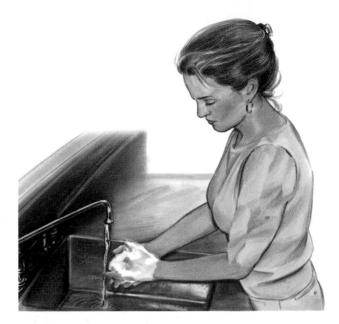

Figure 2. Wash your hands well with soap and lots of water after taking off your gloves.

Important

Use a hand sanitizer if you can't wash your hands with soap and water. Rub your hands well to loosen germs and then allow the sanitizer to air dry.

Universal Precautions

Definitions and Key Facts

This section is based on recommendations of the Centers for Disease Control and Prevention (CDC). Universal precautions are intended to protect you and your coworkers. For best protection, you should treat everyone's blood as if it were infected.

Body fluids, such as blood, saliva, and urine, can sometimes carry germs that cause diseases. Personal protective equipment (PPE) protects you. PPE includes

- Gloves to protect your hands from blood and other body fluids
- Eye protection, if the injured person is bleeding, to protect your eyes from blood and other body fluids
- Mask to protect you when you give breaths

Actions for Universal Precautions

Step	Action
1	Wear personal protective equipment whenever necessary.
2	Place all disposable equipment that has touched blood or body fluids containing blood in a biohazard waste bag (or as required by your workplace).
3	To dispose of the biohazard waste bag, follow your company's plan for disposing of hazardous waste.
4	Wash your hands well with soap and lots of water after properly taking off your gloves.

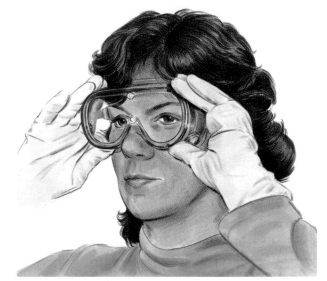

Figure 3. Wear protective gloves whenever you give first aid and wear eye protection if the ill or injured person is bleeding.

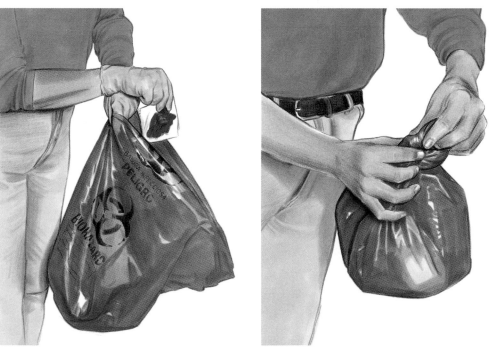

Figure 4. Place all disposable equipment that has touched body fluids, including the gloves you wore, in a biohazard waste bag if one is available. Dispose of the bag according to company policy.

Important	**Latex allergies** are common and can be serious. Some rescuers and ill or injured people may be allergic to latex. Use protective gloves that don't contain latex, such as vinyl gloves, whenever possible.
	If you or the ill or injured person has a latex allergy, do not use gloves that contain latex.

Exposure to Blood

Definitions and Key Facts	Bloodborne diseases are caused by germs. A rescuer may catch a disease if germs in someone else's blood or body fluids enter the rescuer's body, often through the rescuer's mouth or eye or a cut on the skin. To be safe, rescuers should wear personal protective equipment—gloves and eye shields (goggles)—to keep from touching the injured person's blood or body fluids.

Three examples of bloodborne diseases are

- Human immunodeficiency virus (HIV), the virus that causes AIDS
- Hepatitis B
- Hepatitis C

Actions: Exposure to Blood

Step	Action
1	If you are wearing gloves, take them off.
2	Immediately wash your hands and the contact area with soap and lots of water.
3	If body fluids have splattered in your eyes, nose, or the inside of your mouth, rinse these areas with lots of water.
4	Tell your company's emergency response program supervisor what happened as soon as possible. Then contact a healthcare professional.

Taking Off Gloves (*Skill You Will Demonstrate)

Definitions and Key Facts	When you give first aid, the outside of your gloves may touch blood or other body fluids. Take your gloves off without touching the outside of the gloves with your bare hands.

Action:
Taking Off Gloves

Step	Action
1	Grip 1 glove on the outside of the glove near the cuff and peel it down until it comes off inside out.
2	Cup it with your other (gloved) hand.
3	Place 2 fingers of your bare hand inside the cuff of the glove that is still on your hand.
4	Peel that glove off so that it comes off inside out, with the first glove inside it.
5	If there is blood on the gloves, dispose of the gloves properly. • Put them in a biohazard waste bag or as required by your workplace. • If you do not have a biohazard waste bag, put the gloves in a plastic bag that can be sealed before you dispose of it.
6	Wash your hands after you give first aid so that you don't spread germs.

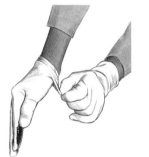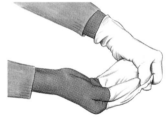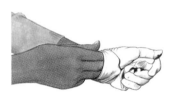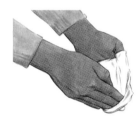

Figure 5. Proper removal of protective gloves—without touching the outside of the gloves.

FYI

Use waterless hand sanitizers only if you do not have immediate access to soap and water. Wash your hands with soap and lots of water as soon as you can.

3. Phoning for Help

What You Will Learn In this section we'll cover

- When to Phone for Help
- How to Phone for Help

Definitions and Key Facts

The American Heart Association adult **Chain of Survival** shows the most important actions needed to treat life-threatening emergencies in adults. The first link in this adult Chain of Survival is to recognize the emergency and phone an emergency number to get help. This section will teach you how and when to phone.

Every place of business should have a plan for emergency response. This tells workers who, how, and sometimes when to phone for help in an emergency.

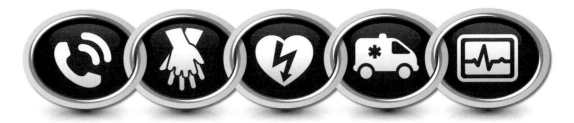

Figure 6. The AHA adult Chain of Survival. The first link in the adult chain is to recognize the emergency and phone for help. This is followed by early CPR with emphasis on compressions, rapid AED use, effective advanced care, and coordinated care afterward.

When to Phone for Help

Definitions and Key Facts

Your company may have some instructions about when you should phone the emergency response number (or 911). In this Student Workbook you'll learn when to phone for help in specific emergencies.

Action: Assess When to Phone for Help

As a general rule, you should phone the emergency response number (or 911) and ask for help whenever

- Someone is seriously ill or injured
- You are not sure what to do in an emergency

Here are some examples of someone who is seriously ill or injured. The person

- Does not respond to voice or touch
- Has chest discomfort
- Has signs of stroke
- Has a problem breathing
- Has a severe injury or burn
- Has a seizure
- Suddenly can't move a part of the body
- Has received an electric shock
- Has been exposed to poison

If someone tries to commit suicide or is assaulted, phone the emergency response number (or 911) regardless of the person's condition.

Definitions and Key Facts

Your company's policy may be to call security, a response team, or the local EMS system number (in many communities this is 911).

Know your phone system. Do you need to dial 9 to get an outside line before you dial your emergency response number (or 911)? You should know your company's emergency response number and phone that number whenever you need help.

Write the emergency response number on your Quick Reference Guide, in the first aid kit, and near the telephone. You should also write it here.

Write your emergency response number here:

_____

Action: How to Phone for Help

If you are	Then you should
Alone	1. Yell for help while you start to check the ill or injured person.
	2. If no one answers your yell and immediate care isn't needed
	a. Leave for a moment while you phone your emergency response number (or 911)
	b. Get the first aid kit and automated external defibrillator (AED), if available
	3. Return to the ill or injured person.
With others	1. Stay with the ill or injured person and be prepared to give first aid or CPR if you know how.
	2. Send someone else to phone your emergency response number (or 911) and get the first aid kit and AED if available.

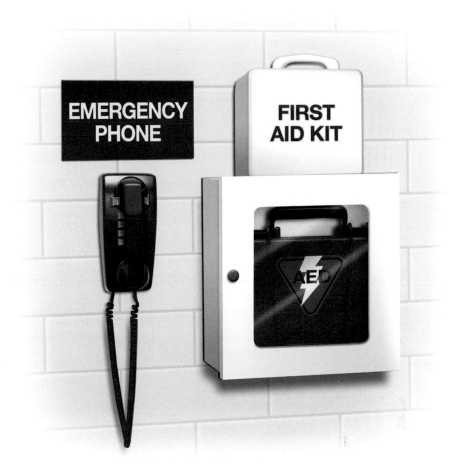

Figure 7. Know the location of the nearest phone to use in an emergency.

Important	Answering all of a dispatcher's questions is important to getting help to you as fast as possible. Do not hang up until the dispatcher tells you to. Answering the dispatcher's questions won't delay the arrival of help.
FYI: Emergency Dispatchers	When you phone for help, the emergency dispatcher may be able to tell you how to do CPR, use an AED, or give first aid.

4. Finding the Problem (*Skill You Will Demonstrate)

What You Will Learn	In this section we'll cover the steps of finding the problem.
Definitions and Key Facts	After you check the scene to be sure it is safe, you must find out what the problem is before you give first aid. Learn to look for problems in order of importance. First look for problems that may be life threatening. Then look for other problems.

Someone who "responds" moves, speaks, blinks, or otherwise reacts to you when you tap him and ask, "Are you OK?" Someone who doesn't "respond" does nothing when you tap him and ask if he's OK.

A person who gasps usually appears to be drawing air in very quickly. He may open his mouth and move the jaw, head, or neck. Gasps may appear forceful or weak, and some time may pass between gasps since they usually happen at a slow rate. The gasp may sound like a snort, snore, or groan. Gasping is not regular or normal breathing. It is a sign of cardiac arrest in someone who doesn't respond.

Action: Find the Problem

The following steps will help you find out what the problem is. They are listed in order of importance, with the most important step listed first.

1. When you arrive at the scene, **check the scene to be sure it is safe.** As you walk toward the ill or injured person, try to look for signs of the cause of the problem.

2. Check whether the person responds. **Tap the person and shout, "Are you OK?"**

   - A person who responds and is awake may be able to answer your questions. Tell the person you're there to help, ask permission to help, and ask what the problem is.
   - A person may only be able to move, moan, or groan when you tap him and shout. If so phone or send someone to phone your emergency response number (or 911) and get the first aid kit and AED.

3. **Next, check if the person is breathing.** If the person isn't breathing or is only gasping, begin CPR and use an AED if you know how.

   If you don't know CPR and you aren't learning it today, give Hands-Only™ CPR. To learn about Hands-Only CPR, go to **handsonlycpr.org.**

4. **Next, look for any obvious signs of injury, such as bleeding, broken bones, burns, or bites.** (You will learn about each of these problems later.)

5. **Finally, look for medical information jewelry.** This tells you if the person has a serious medical condition.

FYI

The muscles at the back of the throat relax in a person who does not respond. When the muscles relax, the tongue may fall back and block the airway. A person with a blocked airway cannot breathe.

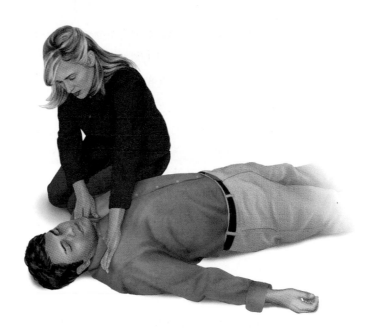

Figure 8. Check if the person responds. Tap him and shout, "Are you OK?"

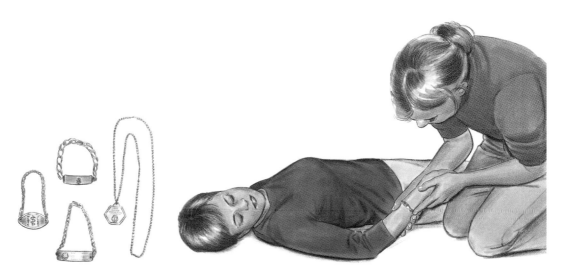

Figure 9. Look for medical information jewelry.

5. After the Emergency

What You Will Learn In this section we'll cover privacy and what you should do after the emergency.

Definitions and Key Facts

As a first aid rescuer you will learn private things about your coworkers, such as their medical condition. Give all information about an ill or injured person to EMS rescuers and your company's emergency response program supervisor. You may also need to fill out a report for your company.

You must not share this information with other coworkers. Keep private things private.

Actions:
Privacy

- Give all information about an ill or injured person to EMS rescuers.
- Fill out the company's report or forms.
- Protect the ill or injured person's privacy.

Sample First Aid Kit

The following table lists sample first aid kit contents. This is a kit that follows ANSI standards. Different workplaces may have different requirements.

Item	Minimum Size or Volume	Quantity per Package	Unit Package Size
List of important local emergency telephone numbers, including police, fire department, EMS, and poison control center*			
Absorbent compress	32 sq. in.	1	1
Adhesive bandage	1 in. × 3 in.	16	1
Adhesive tape	2.5 yd. (total)	1 or 2	1 or 2
Antibiotic treatment	0.14 fl. oz.	6	1
Antiseptic swab	0.14 fl. oz.	10	1
Antiseptic wipe	1 in. × 1 in.	10	1
Antiseptic towelette	24 sq. in.	10	1
Bandage compress (2 in.)	2 in. × 36 in.	4	1
Bandage compress (3 in.)	3 in. × 60 in.	2	1
Bandage compress (4 in.)	4 in. × 72 in.	1	1
Burn dressing	4 in. × 4 in.	1	1 or 2
Burn treatment	1/32 oz.	6	1
CPR barrier		1	1 or 2
Cold pack	4 in. × 5 in.	1	2
Eye covering, with means of attachment	2.9 sq. in.	2	1
Eye/skin wash	4 fl. oz. total	1	2
Gloves		2 pairs	1 or 2
Roller bandage (4 in.)	4 in. × 4 yd.	1	1
Roller bandage (2 in.)	2 in. × 4 yd.	2	1
Sterile pad	3 in. × 3 in.	4	1
Triangular bandage	40 in. × 40 in. × 56 in.	1	1
Heartsaver First Aid Quick Reference Guide*			

*Items meet the ANSI Z308.1-2009 standard, except those marked with an asterisk.

Question	Your Notes
1. When you are providing first aid you should a. wear personal protective equipment (PPE). b. only wear PPE if the person is someone you do not know. c. not be concerned about PPE if you wash your hands. d. use cloth gloves to protect your hands.	
2. When you phone for help, you should stay on the line with the dispatcher until a. people with more advanced training arrive. b. the dispatcher tells you it's OK to hang up.	
3. After giving first aid, you a. can talk about what happened with anyone you want. b. cannot discuss anything with coworkers; you must keep private things private. c. can speak to a reporter about the incident. d. can discuss the incident with your immediate coworkers only.	

(continued)

(continued)

Question	Your Notes

4. You should wash your hands for at least
 	
    a. 10 seconds.
 	
    b. 15 seconds.
 	
    c. 20 seconds.
 	
    d. 3 minutes.	

5. When assessing the scene, you should consider which of the following: (circle all that apply)
 	
    a. Danger to yourself and others
 	
    b. How many people are injured or ill
 	
    c. Where the location is
 	
    d. Where the nearest telephone is	

6. You should replace any supplies you use from the first aid kit. True False	

Answers: 1. a, 2. b, 3. b, 4. c, 5. All, 6. True

Part 2: Medical Emergencies

What You Will Learn	You'll learn how to provide first aid for medical emergencies.

Definitions and Key Facts	At any time, especially during medical emergencies, someone may need CPR. See if the person needs CPR. If he does, give CPR. If you don't know how, give Hands-Only CPR.

Topics Covered	■ Breathing Problems
	■ Choking in an Adult
	■ Allergic Reactions
	■ Heart Attack
	■ Fainting
	■ Diabetes and Low Blood Sugar
	■ Stroke
	■ Seizure
	■ Shock

1. Breathing Problems

What You Will Learn	In this section we'll cover
	■ General Breathing Problems
	■ Assembling and Using an Inhaler
	■ How to Help Someone With Breathing Problems

General Breathing Problems

Definitions and Key Facts	Someone may develop mild or severe blockage of the air passages. Someone having a heart attack, having a stroke, or experiencing certain injuries may also have breathing problems.

Signs

You can tell if someone is having trouble breathing if the person

- Is breathing very fast or very slowly
- Is having trouble with every breath
- Has noisy breathing—you hear a sound or whistle as the air enters or leaves the lungs
- Can only make sounds or speak no more than a few words at a time in between breaths, although the person is trying to say more

Many people with medical conditions, such as asthma, know about their conditions and carry inhaler medicine that can make them feel better within minutes of using it. Sometimes people have so much trouble breathing they need help using their inhalers. You may need to help them.

Assembling and Using an Inhaler

Definitions and Key Facts

Inhalers are made up of 2 parts: the medicine canister and the mouthpiece. A spacer can be attached that makes it easier for the person with the breathing problem to inhale all the medicine.

When someone has trouble breathing, she may panic. For this reason, you should be ready to assemble the inhaler and help her use it.

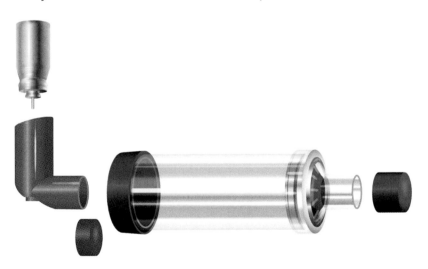

Figure 10. The parts of an inhaler: medicine canister, mouthpiece, and spacer.

Actions

Follow these steps to assemble and use an inhaler:

Step	Action
1	Shake the medicine.
2	Put the medicine canister into the mouthpiece.
3	Remove the cap from the mouthpiece.

(continued)

20

(continued)

Step	Action
4	Attach a spacer if there is one available and if you know how.
5	Tilt the person's head back slightly and have him breathe out slowly.
6	Put the inhaler or spacer in the person's mouth.
7	Push down on the top of the medicine canister. Have the person breathe in slowly and deeply as you push down.
8	Have the person hold his breath for 10 seconds, and then breathe out slowly.

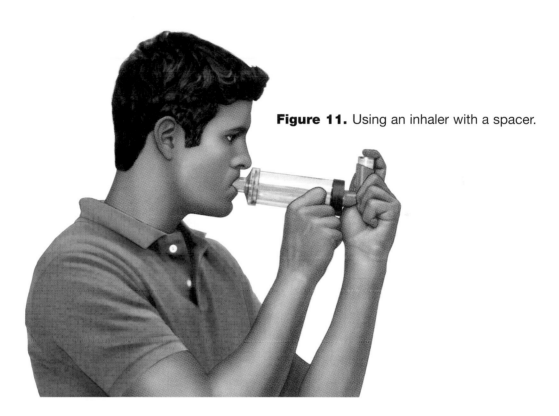

Figure 11. Using an inhaler with a spacer.

How to Help Someone With Breathing Problems

Actions

Follow these steps for someone who is having breathing problems:

Step	Action
1	Make sure the scene is safe.
2	Ask the person if she has medicine. If she needs her medicine but is too sick to get it herself, get it for her.
3	Ask the person if you have the right medicine.
4	Assemble and use the inhaler.

(continued)

(continued)

Step	Action
5	Phone the your emergency response number (or 911) if • The person has no medicine • The person does not get better after using her medicine • The person's breathing gets worse, the person has trouble speaking, or the person stops responding
6	Stay with the person until someone with more advanced training arrives and takes over.
7	See if the person needs CPR. If he does, give CPR. If you don't know how, give Hands-Only CPR.

2. Choking in an Adult

What You Will Learn

In this section we'll cover

- Mild vs Severe Choking
- How to Help a Choking Adult
- How to Help a Choking Adult Who Stops Responding

Definitions and Key Facts

Choking is when food or another object gets stuck in the airway in the throat. The object stops air from getting to the lungs.

Some choking is mild and some is severe. If it's severe, act fast. Get the object out so the person can breathe.

Mild vs Severe Choking

Use the following table to figure out if someone has mild or severe choking and what you should do:

If someone	The block in the airway is	And you should
• Can make sounds • Can cough loudly	Mild	• Stand by and let her cough • If worried about her breathing, phone your emergency response number (or 911)

(continued)

(continued)

If someone	The block in the airway is	And you should
• Cannot breathe or • Has a cough that has no sound or • Cannot talk or make a sound or • Makes the choking sign	Severe	• Act quickly • Follow the steps to help a choking adult

FYI:
The Choking Sign

If someone is choking, he might use the choking sign (holding the neck with one or both hands).

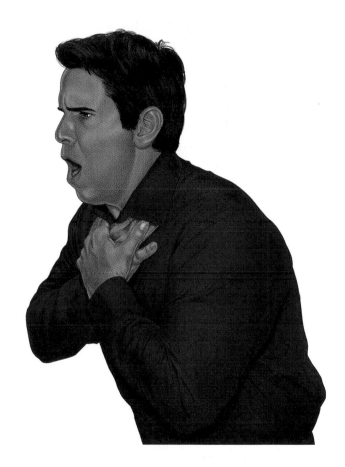

Figure 12. The choking sign: holding the neck with one or both hands.

How to Help a Choking Adult

Definitions and
Key Facts

When someone has severe choking, give thrusts slightly above the belly button. These thrusts are sometimes called the Heimlich maneuver. Like a cough, each thrust pushes air from the lungs. This can help remove an object that is blocking the airway.

**Action:
Help a Choking
Adult**

Follow these steps to help a choking adult:

Step	Action
1	If you think someone is choking, ask, "Are you choking?" If he nods yes, tell him you are going to help.
2	**Get behind him**. Wrap your arms around him so that your hands are in front.
3	**Make a fist** with 1 hand.
4	Put the thumb side of your fist slightly above his belly button and well below the breastbone.
5	**Grasp the fist with your other hand** and give quick upward thrusts into his abdomen.
6	**Give thrusts** until the object is forced out and he can breathe, cough, or talk, or until he stops responding.

Figure 13. Helping someone who is choking.

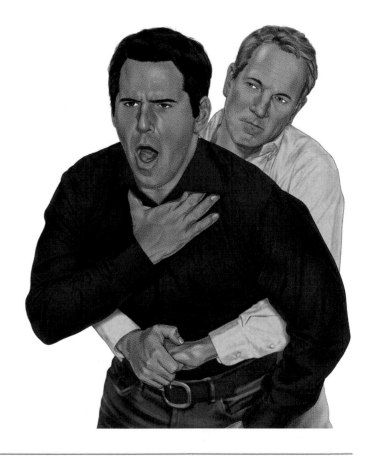

**Action:
Help a Choking
Large Person or
Pregnant Woman**

If someone is choking and is in the late stages of pregnancy or is very large and you can't wrap your arms fully around the waist, give thrusts on the chest, instead of thrusts on the abdomen.

Follow the same steps except for the location where you place your arms and hands. Put your arms under the armpits and your hands on the lower half of the breastbone. Pull straight back to give the chest thrusts.

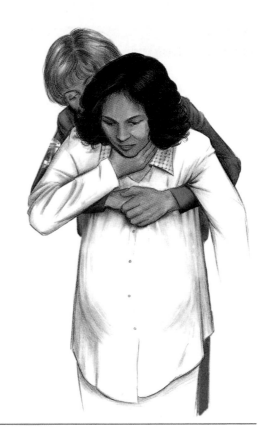

Figure 14. Chest thrusts on a choking large person or pregnant woman.

FYI

Any person who has received thrusts should tell her healthcare provider.

How to Help a Choking Adult Who Stops Responding

Definitions and Key Facts

If you give someone thrusts but can't remove the object blocking the airway, the person will stop responding.

If the person stops responding, follow these steps:

Action

Step	Action
1	Check if he needs CPR. Give it if needed.
2	After each set of 30 compressions, open the airway. If you see an object in the mouth, take it out.
3	Continue CPR until he speaks, moves, or breathes or until someone with more advanced training arrives and takes over.

3. Allergic Reactions

What You Will Learn

In this section we'll cover

- Using Epinephrine Pens (*Skill You Will Demonstrate)
- Mild vs Severe Allergic Reactions

Definitions and Key Facts

Many allergic reactions are mild. Some reactions that seem mild can become severe within minutes.

People can be allergic to many things, including

- Many foods, such as eggs, nuts, chocolate
- Insect stings or bites, especially bee or wasp stings

FYI

Some states and organizations permit first aid rescuers to help people use their epinephrine pens. People who carry epinephrine pens usually know when and how to use them.

You may help give the injection if you are approved to do so by your state regulations and by your company.

Using Epinephrine Pens (*Skill You Will Demonstrate)

Definitions and Key Facts

An epinephrine pen will help someone with a severe allergic reaction breathe more easily. It contains a small amount of medicine that can be injected through clothing. It usually takes several minutes before the medicine starts to work.

The epinephrine injection is given in the side of the thigh.

Actions for an Epinephrine Pen

Step	Action
1	Get the prescribed epinephrine pen.
2	Take off the safety cap. Follow the instructions on the pen.
3	Hold the epinephrine pen in your fist without touching either end because the needle comes out of one end.
4	Push the end with the needle hard against the side of the person's thigh, about halfway between the hip and knee. Give the injection through clothes or on bare skin.
5	Hold the pen in place for about 10 seconds.
6	Remove the needle by pulling the pen straight out.

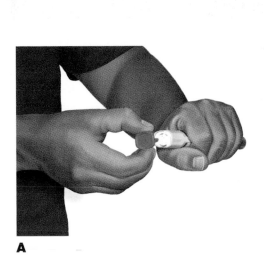
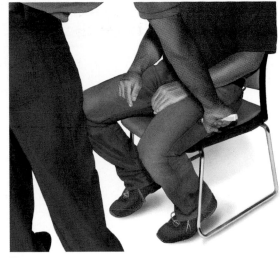

A **B**

Figure 15. Using an epinephrine pen. **A,** Taking off the safety cap. **B,** A rescuer uses the pen.

Mild vs Severe Allergic Reactions

Definitions and Key Facts

Many allergic reactions are mild. Some reactions that seem mild can become severe within minutes.

Signs

The following table shows signs of mild and severe allergic reactions:

Mild Allergic Reaction	Severe Allergic Reaction
• A stuffy nose, sneezing, and itching around the eyes • Itching of the skin • Raised, red rash on the skin (hives)	• Trouble breathing • Swelling of the tongue and face • Signs of shock

Actions for Severe Allergic Reactions

A severe allergic reaction can be life threatening. Follow these steps if you see signs of a severe allergic reaction:

Step	Action
1	Make sure the scene is safe.
2	Phone or send someone to phone your emergency response number (or 911) and get the first aid kit.
3	If the person responds and has an epinephrine pen, help him get it. Ask him to use it.

(continued)

(continued)

Step	Action
4	If he can't use it himself, and if you're allowed, use the epinephrine pen to give him an injection.
5	Rub the injection spot for about 10 seconds.
6	After using the epinephrine pen, dispose of it properly.
7	Note the time of the injection.
8	See if the person needs CPR. If he does, give CPR. If you don't know how, give Hands-Only CPR.

FYI

If possible, save a sample of what caused the reaction.

Important

It's important to dispose of needles correctly so that no one gets stuck. Follow your company's sharps disposal policy. If you don't know what to do, give the needle to someone with more advanced training than you have.

4. Heart Attack

What You Will Learn

In this section we'll cover how to recognize and provide first aid for heart attacks.

Definitions and Key Facts

Heart disease is the single biggest cause of death in the United States.

The first minutes of a heart attack are the most important. This is when the person is likely to get worse and may die. Also many of the treatments for heart attack will be most successful if they are given quickly.

Signs of a Heart Attack

Signs of a heart attack may include

Chest discomfort. Most heart attacks involve discomfort in the center of the chest that lasts more than a few minutes or that goes away and comes back. It can feel like uncomfortable pressure, squeezing, fullness, or pain. If someone has an uncomfortable feeling in the chest, think heart attack.

Discomfort in other areas of the upper body. Symptoms can include pain or discomfort in one or both arms, the back, neck, jaw, or abdomen.

Shortness of breath. This may occur with or without chest discomfort.

Other signs may include cold sweat, nausea, or light-headedness.

Signs in Women, the Elderly, and Diabetics

Women, the elderly, and people with diabetes are more likely to have the less typical signs of a heart attack, such as an ache in the chest, heartburn, or indigestion. They may have an uncomfortable feeling in the back, jaw, neck, or shoulder. They may also complain of shortness of breath or have nausea or vomiting.

Important

Many people won't admit that their discomfort may be caused by a heart attack. People often say

- "I'm too healthy,"
- "I don't want to bother the doctor,"
- "I don't want to frighten my wife," or
- "I'll feel silly if it isn't a heart attack."

If you suspect someone is having a heart attack, act quickly. Don't hesitate, even if the person is uncomfortable admitting his discomfort.

Actions

Follow these steps if someone has any of the signs of a possible heart attack:

Step	Action
1	Make sure the person stays calm and rests.
2	Phone or have someone phone your **emergency response number (or 911).**
3	Ask someone to get the first aid kit and AED if available.
4	If the person has no allergy to aspirin, no serious bleeding, and no signs of a stroke, **give him an aspirin** (either 2 low-dose aspirin or 1 regular).
5	See if the person needs CPR. If he does, give CPR. If you don't know how, give Hands-Only CPR.

Important

It's best if the person doesn't drive himself to the hospital. Stay with him until someone with more advanced training arrives and takes over.

5. Fainting

What You Will Learn

In this section we'll cover what fainting is and how to provide first aid for it.

Definitions and Key Facts

Fainting is a short period when a person stops responding for less than a minute and then seems fine. This is usually caused by not enough blood going to the brain. Seconds before fainting, he may feel dizzy.

Fainting often occurs when the person

- Stands without moving for a long time, especially if the weather is hot
- Has a heart condition
- Suddenly stands after squatting or bending down
- Receives bad news

Actions

Follow these steps if a person is dizzy but still responds:

Step	Action
1	Make sure the scene is safe.
2	Help the person lie flat on the floor.
3	If the person doesn't improve or stops responding, phone your **emergency response number (or 911).**

If a person faints and then starts to respond:

Step	Action
1	Ask the person to continue to lie flat on the floor until he can sit up and feels normal.
2	If the person fell, look for injuries caused by the fall.
3	Phone your **emergency response number (or 911)**.

6. Diabetes and Low Blood Sugar

What You Will Learn

In this section we'll cover how to recognize and provide first aid for low blood sugar in a person with diabetes.

Definitions and Key Facts

Diabetes is a disease that affects levels of sugar in the blood. Too much or too little sugar causes problems. In this course, we're going to address low blood sugar, which can cause someone's behavior to change.

Some diabetics take insulin. Too much insulin can also cause low blood sugar.

Low blood sugar can occur if a person with diabetes has

- Not eaten or is vomiting
- Not eaten enough food for the level of activity
- Injected too much insulin

Signs

Signs of low blood sugar can appear quickly and may include

- A change in behavior, such as confusion or irritability
- Sleepiness or not responding
- Hunger, thirst, or weakness
- Sweating, pale skin color
- A seizure (see the section on seizures)

Actions

Follow these steps if someone is responding and shows signs of low blood sugar:

Step	Action
1	If the person can sit up and swallow, give him something that contains sugar to eat or drink.
2	Have him sit quietly or lie down.
3	Phone or have someone phone your emergency response number (or 911).

FYI

The following list shows what to give a person with diabetes who has low blood sugar. Give foods that contain sugar, such as

- Fruit juice
- Milk
- Sugar
- Honey
- A regular soft drink

It's important to make sure that whatever you give has sugar in it. Diet foods and drinks don't have sugar; chocolate doesn't have enough sugar.

Important

If someone with low blood sugar is unable to sit up and swallow, don't give him anything to eat or drink.

7. Stroke

What You Will Learn

In this section we'll cover how to recognize and provide first aid for stroke.

Definitions and Key Facts

Strokes occur when blood stops flowing to a part of the brain. This can happen if there is bleeding or a blocked blood vessel in the brain. The signs of a stroke are usually very sudden.

New treatments can reduce the damage from a stroke and improve recovery. However, they must be given within the first hours after the first signs of stroke appear. As a result, it's important to recognize the signs of a stroke quickly and get medical care fast.

Signs

The warning signs of stroke are

- Sudden numbness or weakness of the face, arm, or leg, especially on one side of the body
- Sudden confusion, trouble speaking, or trouble understanding
- Sudden trouble seeing in one or both eyes
- Sudden trouble walking, dizziness, loss of balance or coordination
- Sudden, severe headache with no known cause

Actions

Follow these steps if you think someone is having a stroke:

Step	Action
1	Make sure the scene is safe.
2	Phone or ask someone to phone your emergency response number (or 911) and get the first aid kit and an AED if available.
3	Note the time when the signs of stroke first appeared.
4	See if the person needs CPR. If he does, give CPR. If you don't know how, give Hands-Only CPR.

8. Seizure

What You Will Learn

In this section we'll cover how to recognize and provide first aid for seizures.

Definitions and Key Facts

A seizure is abnormal electrical activity in the brain. Most seizures stop within a few minutes. A medical condition called epilepsy often causes seizures. Not all seizures are due to epilepsy. Some seizures happen when the heart suddenly stops beating. Seizures can also be caused by

- Head injury
- Low blood sugar
- Heat-related injury
- Poisons

The person may bite his tongue during a seizure. You can give first aid for that injury after the seizure stops. After a seizure it is not unusual for the person to be confused or get sleepy.

Signs

During some types of seizures, the person may

- Lose muscle control
- Fall to the ground
- Jerk arms, legs, or other parts of the body
- Stop responding

Actions

During a seizure you should follow these steps:

Step	Action
1	Make sure the scene is safe.
2	**Protect the person** by • Moving furniture or other objects out of the way • Placing a small pad or towel under the person's head if it's easy to do so
3	Phone or have someone phone your company's **emergency response number (or 911).**

After a seizure, follow these steps:

Step	Action
1	**See if the person needs CPR.** If he does, give CPR. If you don't know how, give Hands-Only CPR.
2	**Stay with the person** until someone with more advanced training arrives and takes over.
3	If the person is vomiting or has fluids in his mouth and you think the person doesn't have a head, neck, or spine injury, **roll him to his side.**

| **Important** | There are many myths about what to do when someone has a seizure. Some actually tell you to do things that hurt the person who's seizing. (For example, putting a wooden spoon in the mouth can block breathing.) Follow these tables to provide the best and safest first aid. |

9. Shock

| **What You Will Learn** | In this section we'll cover how to recognize and provide first aid for shock. |

| **Definitions and Key Facts** | Shock develops when there is not enough blood flowing to the cells of the body. Someone with shock may stop responding. In adults shock is most often present if someone |

- Loses a lot of blood that you may or may not be able to see
- Has a severe heart attack
- Has a severe allergic reaction

| **Signs** | A person in shock may |

- Feel weak, faint, or dizzy
- Feel nauseous or thirsty
- Have pale or grayish skin
- Act restless, agitated, or confused
- Be cold and clammy to the touch

Actions

Step	Action
1	Make sure the scene is safe.
2	Phone or send someone to phone your company's emergency response number (or 911) and get the first aid kit and AED.
3	Help the person **lie on her back.**
4	**Cover the person in shock** to keep her warm.
5	**See if the person needs CPR**. If she does, give CPR. If you don't know how, give Hands-Only CPR.

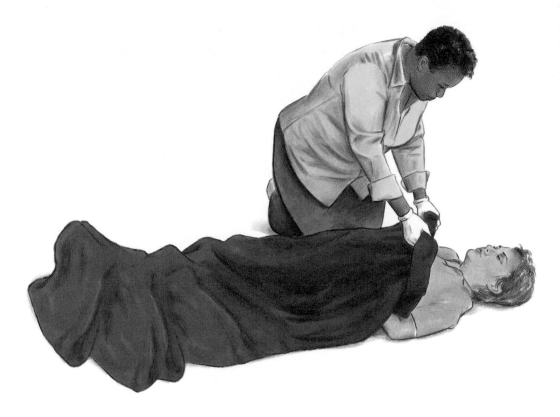

Figure 16. Cover a person in shock.

Review Questions: Medical Emergencies

Question	Your Notes
1. When giving abdominal thrusts to an adult who is choking, you should a. place your hands near the throat. b. place your hands near the left side of the lower abdomen. c. put the thumb side of your fist slightly above her navel (belly button) and well below the breastbone.	

(continued)

(continued)

Question	Your Notes
2. Signs of a severe allergic reaction include trouble breathing, swelling of the face and tongue, and the person may stop responding. True False	

3. A person with a _____ is usually awake and can talk but may have an uncomfortable feeling, such as pain or pressure, in the chest.
 	
  a. stroke
 	
  b. seizure
 	
  c. heart attack	

4. The warning signs of _____ include sudden numbness or weakness of the face, arm, or leg, especially on one side of the body.
 	
  a. fainting
 	
  b. stroke
 	
  c. heart attack
 	
  d. seizure	

5. If someone with low blood sugar is responding and can sit up and swallow, give her something that contains sugar to eat or drink. True False	

Answers: 1. c, 2. True, 3. c, 4. b, 5. True

Part 3: Injury Emergencies

What You Will Learn	You'll learn how to provide first aid for injury emergencies.
Definitions and Key Facts	At any time, especially during injury emergencies, someone may need CPR. See if the person needs CPR. If he does, give CPR. If you don't know how, give Hands-Only CPR.
Topics Covered	■ Bleeding You Can See ■ Wounds ■ Bleeding You Can't See ■ Head, Neck, and Spine Injuries ■ Broken Bones and Sprains ■ Burns and Electrical Injuries

1. Bleeding You Can See

What You Will Learn	In this section we'll cover ■ How to Stop Bleeding (*Skill You Will Demonstrate) ■ Bandaging (*Skill You Will Demonstrate) ■ Using Tourniquets

How to Stop Bleeding (*Skill You Will Demonstrate)

Definitions and Key Facts	Bleeding often looks worse than it is. When a large blood vessel is cut or torn, the person can lose a lot of blood within minutes. However, you can stop most bleeding with pressure. If the injured person can help you, ask him to put direct pressure on the wound while you put on your personal protective equipment (PPE). A dressing is a wound covering used to stop bleeding. It helps prevent infection. A dressing can be a gauze pad or any other clean piece of cloth or even a gloved hand.

Phone or ask someone to phone your emergency response number (or 911) if

- There is a lot of bleeding
- You cannot stop the bleeding
- You see signs of shock
- You suspect a head, neck, or spine injury
- You are not sure what to do

Actions for Bleeding You Can See

Take the following actions to stop bleeding that you can see:

Step	Action
1	Make sure the scene is safe. Get the first aid kit. Wear PPE.
2	Put a dressing on the wound. Apply **direct pressure on the dressing.** Use the flat part of your fingers or the palm of your hand.
3	If the bleeding does not stop, **add more dressings** on top of the first and **press harder**.
4	Keep **pressure** on the wound **until it stops bleeding**.
5	If you can't keep pressure on the wound, wrap a bandage firmly over the dressing to hold the dressing in place.

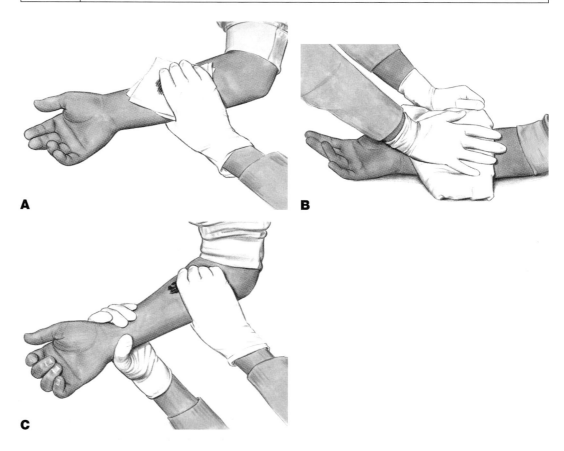

A

B

C

Figure 17. A dressing can be a gauze pad or pads (**A**) or any other clean piece of cloth (**B**). If you do not have a dressing, use your gloved hand (**C**).

FYI: **Multiple Dressings and Antibiotic Creams**	Small wounds heal better and with less infection if an antibiotic ointment or cream is used. Apply antibiotic ointment or cream and then a clean dressing, but only if the wound is a small scrape or surface cut and only if the person doesn't have any allergies to the antibiotic.
Important: **Minor Cuts and Scrapes**	If the cut or scrape is minor, wash the area with lots of clean water to get the wound clean before applying the dressings. You'll use less direct pressure to stop the bleeding for a minor cut or scrape than for a major cut or scrape.

Bandaging (*Skill You Will Demonstrate)

Definitions and Key Facts	A bandage is material used to protect or cover an injured body part. A bandage may also help keep pressure on the wound.

Action

Step	Action
1	Make sure the scene is safe. Get the first aid kit and wear PPE.
2	Use direct pressure, with gauze pads/dressings if available, to stop any bleeding.
3	Apply the bandage over the dressings.

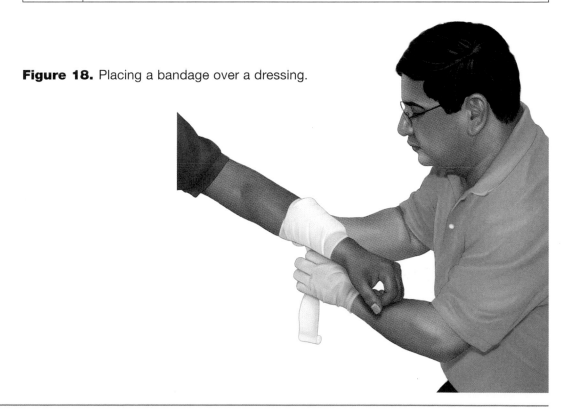

Figure 18. Placing a bandage over a dressing.

Using Tourniquets

Definitions and Key Facts	If an arm or leg has severe bleeding and you can't stop the bleeding with direct pressure, you can use a tourniquet.

The best tourniquets are premade, or manufactured, ones. If you don't have one, you can make a tourniquet out of a piece of cloth and a windlass, essentially a stick-like object used to tighten the tourniquet.

If you apply the tourniquet correctly, it will cause pain as it stops the bleeding. |

Action: Use a Premade Tourniquet

The following steps apply to a premade tourniquet:

Step	Action
1	Make sure the scene is safe. Phone your emergency response number (or 911). Wear PPE.
2	Place the tourniquet 2 inches above the injury, if possible.
3	Tighten the tourniquet until the bleeding stops.
4	Note what time you put the tourniquet on.
5	Get medical help as soon as possible.
6	Leave the tourniquet on until someone with more advanced training takes over.

Important

Once you have the tourniquet in place, leave it alone until someone with more advanced training arrives and takes over.

Action: Make and Use a Tourniquet

If you need to make a tourniquet, follow the steps in this table. Then apply the tourniquet the same way as you would for a premade one.

Step	Action
1	Make sure the scene is safe. Wear PPE.
2	Fold a cloth or bandage so that it's long and at least 1 inch wide.
3	Wrap the bandage 2 inches above the injury, if possible.
4	Tie the ends of the bandage around a stick (or something similar to a stick).
5	Turn the stick to tighten the tourniquet.
6	Continue tightening until the bleeding stops.

(continued)

(continued)

Step	Action
7	Secure the stick so the tourniquet stays tight.
8	Note what time the tourniquet was placed.
9	Get medical help as soon as possible.

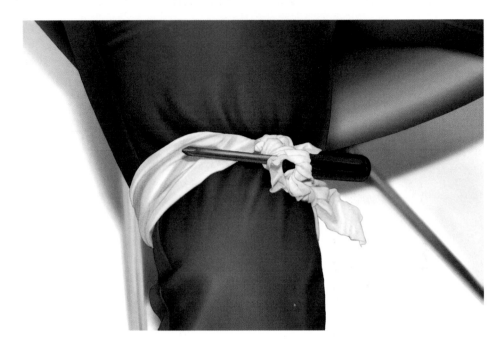

Figure 19. A tourniquet applied to a leg.

FYI

Most first aid kits have a triangular bandage. This is ideal for making a tourniquet.

Important

Leave all dressings on as you add more.

2. Wounds

What You Will Learn

In this section we'll cover

- Bleeding From the Nose
- Bleeding From the Mouth
- Tooth Injuries
- Eye Injuries
- Penetrating and Puncturing Objects
- Amputation

Definitions and Key Facts	With nosebleeds it's sometimes hard to tell how much bleeding there is because the injured person often swallows some of the blood. This may cause the person to vomit.

Actions

Follow these steps when giving first aid to a person with a nosebleed:

Step	Action
1	Make sure the scene is safe. Get the first aid kit. Wear PPE.
2	**Press both sides of the nostrils** while the **person** sits and **leans forward.**
3	Place **constant pressure** on both sides of the nostrils for a few minutes until the bleeding stops.
4	If bleeding continues, press harder.
5	Phone your emergency response number (or 911) if • You can't stop the bleeding in about 15 minutes • The bleeding is heavy, such as gushing blood • The person has trouble breathing

Important

People are sometimes misinformed about the best way to stop a nosebleed. The correct way to help someone with a nosebleed is to follow the steps outlined in the table.

Figure 20. Press on both sides of the nostrils.

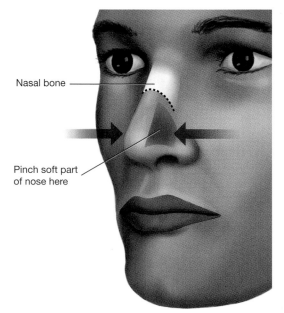

Nasal bone

Pinch soft part of nose here

Definitions and Key Facts

You can usually stop bleeding from the mouth with pressure.

Bleeding from the mouth can be serious if blood or broken teeth block the airway and cause breathing problems or if you can't reach the bleeding area.

Actions

Follow these steps when giving first aid to a person with bleeding from the mouth:

Step	Action
1	Make sure that the scene is safe. Get the first aid kit. Wear PPE.
2	If you can easily reach the bleeding, **apply pressure to the area with dressings.**
3	Phone or ask someone to phone your emergency response number (or 911) if • You can't stop the bleeding • The person has trouble breathing

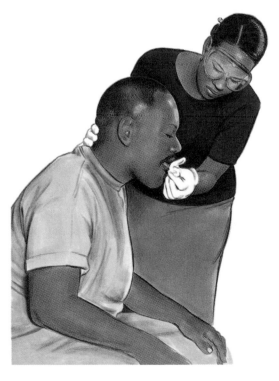

Figure 21. If the bleeding is from the tongue, lip, or cheek, press the bleeding area with sterile gauze or a clean cloth.

Definitions and Key Facts

A person with a mouth injury may have broken, loose, or knocked-out teeth. This can be a choking hazard.

Actions for Tooth Injuries

Follow these steps when giving first aid to a person with a tooth injury:

Step	Action
1	Make sure the scene is safe. Get the first aid kit. Wear PPE.
2	Check the mouth for any missing teeth, loose teeth, or parts of teeth.
3	Clean the wound with saline or clean water.
4	If a tooth is loose, have the person bite down on a piece of gauze to keep the tooth in place and call a dentist.
5	If a tooth is chipped, gently clean the injured area and call a dentist.
6	Apply pressure with gauze to stop any bleeding at the empty tooth socket.
7	If a tooth has come out, put the tooth in a cup of milk or clean water and immediately take the injured person and tooth to a dentist or emergency department.
8	Tell the person to talk with a dentist if a tooth changes color after an injury.

Important

Hold the tooth by the crown, not the root (the part that was in the gums). There may be ligaments on the tooth that will help reattach the tooth.

Keep the tooth out of the mouth.

Figure 22. Hold the tooth by the crown.

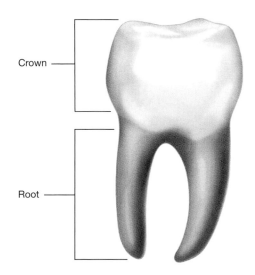

Crown

Root

Definitions and Key Facts

Eye injuries may happen

- With a direct hit or punch to the eye or the side of the head
- When a ball or other object directly hits the eye
- When a high-speed object, such as a BB gun pellet, hits the eye
- When a stick or other sharp object punctures the eye
- When a small object, such as a piece of dirt, gets in the eye

Signs

Signs of an eye injury include

- Pain
- Trouble seeing
- Bruising
- Bleeding
- Redness, swelling

Actions

Follow these steps for eye injuries:

Step	Action
1	Make sure the scene is safe. Get the first aid kit. Wear PPE.
2	Phone or ask someone to phone your emergency response number (or 911) if the eye is hit hard or punctured. Tell the person to keep her eyes closed.
3	If there is an irritant, such as sand, in the eye, use water to rinse the eye.
4	If the irritant does not come out or if the person is in extreme pain, phone or ask someone to phone your emergency response number (or 911). Tell the person to keep her eyes closed.

Penetrating and Puncturing Objects

Definitions and Key Facts

An object such as a knife or sharp stick can wound a person by penetrating the body or puncturing the skin. Leave the object in place until a healthcare provider can treat the injury.

Actions

Follow these steps when giving first aid to a person with an injury from a puncturing or penetrating object:

Step	Action
1	Make sure the scene is safe. Get the first aid kit. Wear PPE.
2	Phone or ask someone to phone your **emergency response number (or 911).**
3	**Stop any bleeding you can see.**
4	Try to keep the injured person from moving.

Important

Leave penetrating objects in.

If a person is injured and a sharp object, such as a nail or a knife, remains partly stuck in the body, leave it in the body. Taking it out may cause more damage.

Amputation

Definitions and Key Facts

If a part of the body, such as a finger, toe, hand, or foot is cut off (amputated), save the body part because doctors may be able to reattach it. You can preserve a detached body part at room temperature, but it will be in a better condition to be reattached if you keep it cool.

Actions

Follow these steps to protect an amputated part:

Step	Action
1	Rinse the amputated part with clean water.
2	Cover or wrap the amputated part with a clean dressing.
3	If it will fit, place the amputated part in a watertight plastic bag.
4	Place that bag in another container with ice or ice and water; label it with the injured person's name, date, and time.
5	Make sure it is sent to the hospital with the injured person.

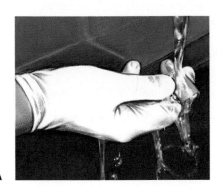
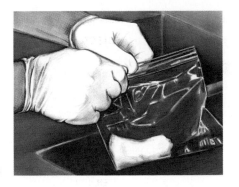
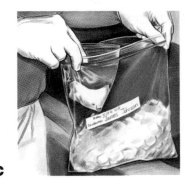

A   **B**   **C**

Figure 23. A, If you can find the amputated part, rinse it with clean water. **B,** If it will fit, place the wrapped part in a watertight plastic bag. **C,** Place that bag in another labeled bag.

Important	Never place the amputated body part directly on ice or in water because the ice or water may damage it.

Actions for Amputation

Follow these steps when giving first aid to a person with an amputation:

Step	Action
1	Make sure the scene is safe. Get the first aid kit and AED. Wear PPE.
2	Phone or ask someone to phone your emergency response number (or 911).
3	Stop the bleeding from the injured area with pressure. **You will have to press for a long time with very firm pressure to stop the bleeding.**
4	If you find the **amputated part, protect it.**
5	Stay with the injured person until someone with more advanced training arrives and takes over.

3. Bleeding You Can't See

What You Will Learn

In this section we'll cover when to suspect bleeding you can't see and how to provide first aid for bleeding you can't see.

Definitions and Key Facts

An injury inside the body may be minor or severe.

Being hit hard in the chest or abdomen or falling can cause bleeding inside the body. You may not see physical signs of this bleeding, or you may see a bruise.

Signs

Suspect bleeding you can't see if a person has

- An injury from a car crash, from being hit by a car, or after a fall from a height
- An injury to the abdomen or chest (including bruises such as seat belt marks)
- Sports injuries such as slamming into other people or being hit with a ball
- Pain in the chest or abdomen after an injury
- Shortness of breath after an injury
- Coughed-up or vomited blood after an injury
- Signs of shock without bleeding that you can see
- A knife or gunshot wound

Actions

Follow these steps when giving first aid to a person who may have bleeding you can't see:

Step	Action
1	Make sure that the scene is safe. Get the first kit and AED. Wear PPE.
2	Phone or ask someone to phone your emergency response number (or 911).
3	Have the person lie down and keep still.
4	Check for signs of shock.
5	See if the person needs CPR. If he does, give CPR. If you don't know how, give Hands-Only CPR.

4. Head, Neck, and Spine Injuries

What You Will Learn

In this section we'll cover how to recognize and provide first aid for head, neck, and spine injuries.

Definitions and Key Facts for Head Injury

Suspect a head injury if the person

- Fell from a height
- Was hit in the head
- Was injured while diving
- Suffered an electrical injury
- Was involved in a car crash
- Was riding a bicycle or motorbike involved in a crash, and has no helmet or a broken helmet

| Signs of Head Injury | Suspect a head injury if an injured person |

Signs of Head Injury

Suspect a head injury if an injured person

- Does not respond or only moans or moves
- Acts sleepy or confused
- Vomits
- Complains of a headache
- Has trouble seeing
- Has trouble walking or moving any part of the body
- Has a seizure

Definitions and Key Facts for Spine and Neck

The bones of the spine protect the spinal cord. The spinal cord carries messages between the brain and the body.

If the spine is damaged, the spinal cord may be injured. The person may not be able to move her legs or arms and may lose feeling in parts of the body. Some people call this a "broken back."

Important

You may cause further injury to the spinal cord if you bend, twist, or turn the person's head or neck. When you give first aid to someone with a possible spine injury, you must not bend, twist, or turn the head or neck unless it's necessary to provide CPR or if you need to move the person out of danger.

If she is vomiting or has fluids in her mouth, wear PPE and roll her to the side.

Signs of a Neck or Spine Injury

Suspect that the spine bones are broken if an injured person

- Is 65 or older
- Was in a car or bicycle crash
- Has fallen from a height
- Has tingling or weakness in the extremities
- Has pain or tenderness in the neck or back
- Appears to be intoxicated or not fully alert
- Has other painful injuries, especially of the head and neck

Actions for Head, Neck, and Spine Injuries

Follow these steps when giving first aid to a person with a possible head, neck, or spine injury:

Step	Action
1	Make sure that the scene is safe.
2	Phone or ask someone to phone your emergency response number (or 911) and get the first aid kit.
3	Minimize movement of the head and neck.

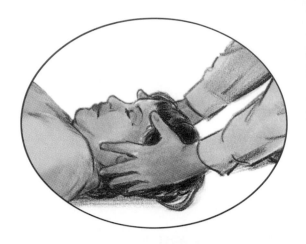

Figure 24. Hold the head and neck to minimize movement.

5. Broken Bones and Sprains

What You Will Learn

In this section we'll cover how to recognize and provide first aid for broken bones and sprains.

Definitions and Key Facts

Joint sprains happen when joints move in directions they're not supposed to go.

Without an x-ray, it may be impossible to tell whether a bone is broken. But you will perform the same actions even if you don't know whether the bone is broken.

Signs

There may be swelling and the joint may turn slightly blue if it is sprained.

Actions

Follow these steps when giving first aid for a person with a possible broken bone or sprain:

Step	Action
1	Make sure that the scene is safe. Get the first aid kit. Wear PPE.
2	Cover any open wound with a clean dressing.
3	Put a **plastic bag** filled with **ice and water on the injured area** with a towel between the ice bag and the skin for up to 20 minutes.
4	Phone or ask someone to phone your emergency response number (or 911) if • There is a large open wound • The injured part is abnormally bent • You're not sure what to do
5	If an injured body part hurts, the person should avoid using it until checked by a healthcare provider.

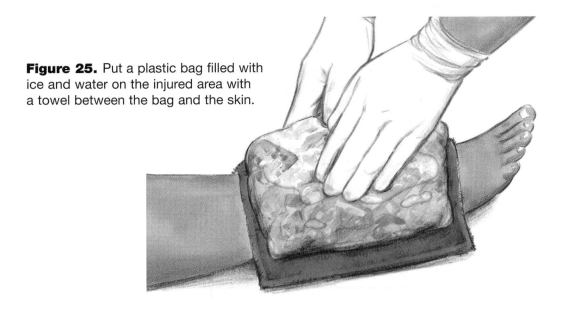

Figure 25. Put a plastic bag filled with ice and water on the injured area with a towel between the bag and the skin.

FYI

You may use a cold pack, but it is not as cold and may not work as well as ice and water.

Don't straighten any body part that's bent or deformed. Don't move a broken bone that has come through the skin.

Splinting (*Skill You May Demonstrate; Optional Practice)

Definitions and Key Facts

A splint keeps an injured body part from moving. In general, healthcare providers apply splints.

At times, you may need to splint an arm or a leg. For example, if you are hiking in the wilderness, you may need to splint an injured arm.

Rolled-up towels, magazines, and pieces of wood can be used as splints.

Actions: Splinting

To splint, follow the actions in the table:

Step	Action
1	Make sure the scene is safe. Get the first aid kit. Wear PPE.
2	To make the splint, use something (such as a magazine) that will keep the arm or leg from moving.
3	Ideally, place the splint so that it extends beyond the injured area and supports the joints above and below the injury.
4	Tie the splint to the injured body part so that it supports the injured area. Use tape, gauze, or cloth to secure it.
5	Make sure that the injured person is checked by a healthcare provider.

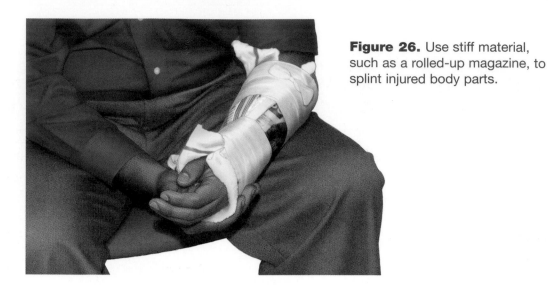

Figure 26. Use stiff material, such as a rolled-up magazine, to splint injured body parts.

FYI	You should be able to put a few fingers between the splint and the injured body part. Do not tie the splint too tightly. This might cause further pain. If you use something hard for the splint, pad the inside of the splint with cloths or dressings, if possible, to keep the person comfortable.
Important	If the injured part is bleeding, apply direct pressure to stop the bleeding and apply a dressing to the wound before applying the splint.
Actions: Self-Splinting an Arm	If you don't have anything to use as a splint, a person can use his other arm to hold the injured one in place. Follow these steps to self-splint an arm:

Step	Action
1	Make sure the scene is safe.
2	Have the injured person place his hand across his chest and hold it in place with his other arm.

Important	Leave bent and deformed body parts in their bent or deformed positions as you apply the splint. If a broken bone has come through the skin, cover the wound with a clean dressing, and splint as needed.

6. Burns and Electrical Injuries

What You Will Learn	In this section we'll cover how to provide first aid for burns and electrical injuries.

Burns

Definitions and Key Facts for Burns

Burns are injuries that can be caused by contact with heat, electricity, or chemicals. Heat burns can be caused by contact with fire, a hot surface, a hot liquid, or steam.

Use cool water on burns. Ice can damage burned areas. If someone with a burn gets too cold, she can get hypothermia (low body temperature).

Actions for Small Burns

Follow these steps to give first aid to a person with a small burn:

Step	Action
1	Make sure the scene is safe. Get the first aid kit. Wear PPE.
2	If the burn area is small, cool it immediately with cold, but not ice-cold, water. Run cold water on the burn until it doesn't hurt.
3	You may cover the burn with a dry, nonstick sterile or clean dressing.

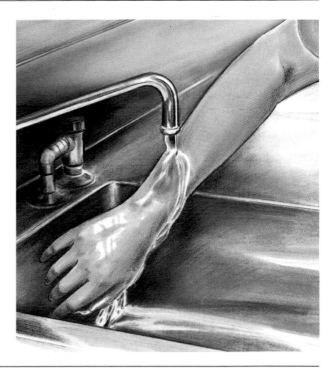

Figure 27. If possible, hold the burned area under cold running water.

Important

Phone or send someone to phone your emergency response number (or 911) if

- There is a fire
- The person has a large burn
- You are not sure what to do

Important	If someone is on fire, put the fire out: Have that person stop, drop, and roll; then cover the person with a wet blanket to put the fire out. Once the fire is out, remove the wet blanket.

Actions for Large Burns	Follow these steps to give first aid to a person with a large burn:

Step	Action
1	Make sure the scene is safe. Get the first aid kit. Phone your emergency response number (or 911).
2	If the person is on fire, put the fire out.
3	Remove jewelry and clothing that is not stuck to the skin.
4	Cover the person with a dry blanket.
5	Check for signs of shock.

FYI	Cover the person with a dry blanket to keep the person warm because once the skin has burned, the person can no longer control body temperature well and often gets cold.

Electrical Injuries

Definitions and Key Facts	Electricity can burn the body on the inside and outside. Electricity can stop breathing or cause a deadly abnormal heart rhythm.

Signs	Electricity may leave only small marks on the body. No one can tell how much damage there is inside the body based on the marks on the outside.

Actions	Follow these steps for giving first aid for an electrical injury:

Step	Action
1	Make sure the scene is safe. Get the first aid kit and AED. Wear PPE.
2	Phone or send someone to phone your emergency response number (or 911).
3	When it is safe to touch the injured person, see if he needs CPR. If he does, give CPR. If you don't know how, give Hands-Only CPR.
4	A healthcare provider should check everyone who has an electrical injury.

Stay clear of the injured person as long as he's in contact with a power source that is on. Electricity can travel from the source through the injured person to you. Turn off the main power switch only if you know how and can safely do so. Once the power is off, you may touch the injured person.

High Voltage

If the electrical injury is caused by high voltage, such as a fallen power line, electricity can travel through everything that touches the power line or source (even a wooden stick). Wait until the power has been turned off to enter the area and provide help.

Important

Many people have heard about different ointments for burns. The only thing you should put on a burn is cool water and clean dressings unless you are given other instructions by a healthcare provider.

Review Questions: Injury Emergencies

Question	Your Notes
1. To help stop bleeding that you can see, put firm pressure on a dressing or bandage over the bleeding area. True False	
2. *Mark an X by the correct response.* A person with a nosebleed should lean ____ forward. ____ backward.	
3. *Mark an X by the correct response.* If a large stick or a knife has been pushed into someone's body, you should ____ remove it as quickly as possible. ____ leave it in and get help.	

(continued)

(continued)

Question	Your Notes
4. If someone falls down and then becomes sleepy or confused, vomits, or complains of a head-ache, the person may have a head injury. True False	
5. As soon as a person twists his ankle, apply a heating pad or heat pack over the injured area for 20 minutes to help reduce swelling. True False	

6. To give first aid for a small burn on the arm, cool the burn with
 	
  a. lukewarm water.
 	
  b. ice directly on the skin.
 	
  c. cold, but not ice-cold, water.	

Answers: **1.** True, **2.** Forward, **3.** Leave it in, **4.** True, **5.** False, **6.** c

Part 4: Environmental Emergencies

What You Will Learn	You'll learn how to provide first aid for environmental emergencies.
Definitions and Key Facts	At any time, especially during environmental emergencies, someone may need CPR. If he does, give CPR. If you don't know how, give Hands-Only CPR.
Topics Covered	■ Bites and Stings ■ Heat-Related Emergencies ■ Cold-Related Emergencies ■ Poison Emergencies

1. Bites and Stings

What You Will Learn	In this section we'll cover ■ Animal and Human Bites ■ Snakebites ■ Insect, Bee, and Spider Bites and Stings ■ Poisonous Spider and Scorpion Bites and Stings ■ Ticks

Animal and Human Bites

Definitions and Key Facts	Although many bites are minor, some may break the skin. When a bite breaks the skin, the wound can bleed and may become infected from the germs in the biter's mouth. Bites that do not break the skin are not usually serious. Be sure to stay away from an animal that is acting strangely.
Actions	Follow these steps to give first aid to a person with an animal or human bite:

Step	Action
1	Make sure the scene is safe. Get the first aid kit. Wear PPE.
2	For animal bites, phone or send someone to phone your emergency response number (or 911).
3	**Clean the wound** with a lot of running water (and soap, if available).
4	**Stop any bleeding** with pressure and dressings.
5	For all bites that break the skin, call a healthcare provider.
6	If there is a bruise or swelling, place a bag of ice and water wrapped in a towel on the bite for up to 20 minutes.

Important

- These animals may carry rabies: cat, dog, skunk, raccoon, fox, bat, or other wild animal.
- If a person is in a room with a bat, contact a healthcare provider.

Snakebites

Definitions and Key Facts

If a snake bites someone, it is helpful to be able to identify the kind of snake. Sometimes you can identify the snake from its bite mark. If you aren't sure whether a snake is poisonous, assume that it is.

Signs of Poisonous Snakebites

- Pain in the bite area that keeps getting worse
- Swelling of the bite area
- Nausea, vomiting, sweating, and weakness

Actions

Follow these steps to give first aid to someone who has been bitten:

Step	Action
1	Make sure the scene is safe. Get the first aid kit. Wear PPE.
2	Ask another adult to move any other people inside or away from the area and phone your emergency response number (or 911).
3	Ask the bitten person to be **still and calm.** Tell him to avoid moving the part of the body that was bitten.
4	**Remove any tight clothing** and jewelry.
5	**Gently wash** the bite area with running water (and soap if available).

Important	Some people have heard about other ways to treat a snakebite, such as sucking out the poison. The correct steps for treating a snakebite are in the table.

Important: Scene Safety and Snakes	<ul><li>When making sure the scene is safe, be very careful around a wounded snake.</li><li>Back away and go around the snake.</li><li>If a snake has been killed or hurt by accident, leave it alone. A snake might bite even when severely hurt or close to death.</li><li>If the snake needs to be moved, use a long-handled shovel. If you don't need to move it, leave it alone.</li></ul>

Insect, Bee, and Spider Bites and Stings

Definitions and Key Facts	Usually insect and spider bites and stings cause only mild pain, itching, and swelling at the bite. Some insect bites can be serious and even fatal if <ul><li>The person bitten has a severe allergic reaction to the bite or sting</li><li>Poison (venom) is injected into the person (for example, from a black widow spider or brown recluse spider)</li></ul>

Actions	Follow these steps to give first aid to someone with a bite or sting:

Step	Action
1	Make sure the scene is safe. Get the first aid kit. Wear PPE.
2	Phone or send someone to phone your emergency response number (or 911) and get the first aid kit if <ul><li>The person has signs of a severe allergic reaction</li><li>The person tells you that she has a severe allergic reaction to insect bites or stings. Get the person's epinephrine pen if she has one.</li></ul>
3	If a **bee** stung the person <ul><li>Look for the stinger. Bees are the only insects that may leave their stingers behind.</li><li>Scrape away the stinger and venom sac by using something with a dull edge, such as a credit card.</li></ul>

(continued)

(continued)

Step	Action
4	**Wash** the bite or sting area with a **lot of running water** (and soap, if possible).
5	Put a **bag of ice and water** wrapped in a towel or cloth over the bite or sting area for up to 20 minutes.
6	Watch the person for at least 30 minutes for signs of an allergic reaction.

Important

Make sure you remove the stinger with something flat and dull that won't squeeze the stinger. Squeezing the venom sac can release more venom (poison).

Poisonous Spider and Scorpion Bites and Stings

Signs

The following are the signs of poisonous spider and scorpion bites and stings. Some of the signs may vary depending on the type of bite or sting.

- Severe pain at the site of the bite or sting
- Muscle cramps
- Headache
- Fever
- Vomiting
- Breathing problems
- Seizures
- Lack of response

Actions

Follow these steps for a spider or scorpion bite or sting:

Step	Action
1	Make sure the scene is safe. Get the first aid kit. Wear PPE.
2	**Phone** your emergency response number (or 911).
3	**Wash** the bite with a lot of **running water (and soap,** if available).
4	Put a **bag of ice and water** wrapped in a towel or cloth on the bite.
5	See if the person needs CPR. If he does, give CPR. If you don't know how, give Hands-Only CPR.

Ticks

Definitions and Key Facts

Ticks are found on animals and in wooded areas. They attach themselves to exposed body parts. Many ticks are harmless. Some carry serious diseases.

If you find a tick, remove it as soon as possible. The longer the tick stays attached to a person, the greater the person's chance of catching a disease.

Actions for Tick Bites

Step	Action
1	Make sure the scene is safe. Get the first aid kit. Wear PPE.
2	**Grab the tick by its mouth or head** as close to the skin as possible with tweezers or a tick-removing device.
3	**Lift the tick straight out** without twisting or squeezing its body. If you lift the tick until the person's skin tents and wait for several seconds, the tick may let go.
4	**Wash** the bite with running water (and soap, if available).
5	See a healthcare provider if you are in an area where tick-borne diseases occur. If possible, place the tick in a plastic bag and give it to the healthcare provider.

Important

Some people have heard about other ways to remove a tick. The correct way to remove a tick is to follow the actions in the table.

2. Heat-Related Emergencies

What You Will Learn

In this section we'll cover

- Heat Cramps
- Heat Exhaustion
- Heat Stroke

Heat Cramps

Definitions and Key Facts

Most heat-related emergencies are caused by vigorous exercise.

Heat cramps are painful muscle spasms, most often in the calves, arms, stomach muscles, and back.

Signs	Signs of heat cramps include muscle cramps, sweating, and headache.

Actions for Heat Cramps

Step	Action
1	Make sure the scene is safe. Get the first aid kit. Wear PPE.
2	Have the person with heat cramps rest and cool off.
3	Have the person drink something that contains sugar and electrolytes, such as juice or a sports drink, or water if the others aren't available.

FYI

Once heat cramp symptoms stop, the person can exercise again. Stretching, icing, and massaging painful muscles may be helpful.

A bag with ice and water and wrapped in a towel may be applied to the sore muscle for up to 20 minutes if the person can tolerate it.

Important

Mild heat-related signs are a warning that the person's condition may get worse unless you take action. Symptoms of heat-related emergencies often increase if left untreated.

Heat Exhaustion

Definitions and Key Facts

Heat exhaustion is a serious condition that often turns into heat stroke. It often occurs when someone exercises in the heat and sweats a lot.

Signs

Signs of heat exhaustion include sweating, nausea, dizziness, vomiting, muscle cramps, feeling faint, and fatigue.

Actions

Follow these steps for heat exhaustion:

Step	Action
1	Make sure the scene is safe. Get the first aid kit. Wear PPE.
2	Phone or ask someone to phone your emergency response number (or 911).
3	Have the person lie down in a cool place.
4	Remove as much of the person's clothing as possible.
5	Cool the person with a cool water spray.

(continued)

(continued)

Step	Action
6	If cool water spray is not available, place cool damp cloths on the neck, armpit, and groin area.
7	Have the person drink something that contains sugar and electrolytes, such as juice or a sports drink, or water if the others aren't available.

Heat Stroke

Definitions and Key Facts

Heat stroke is a very serious condition. It looks similar to heat exhaustion but it is life threatening. You need to act quickly.

Signs

The key signs of heat stroke are confusion, passing out, dizziness, and seizures.

Other signs of heat stroke include nausea, vomiting, muscle cramps, feeling faint, and fatigue.

Actions for Heat Stroke

Step	Action
1	Make sure the scene is safe. Get the first aid kit and AED. Wear PPE.
2	Phone or ask someone to phone your **emergency response number (or 911).**
3	Put the person in **cool water, up to her neck** if possible.
4	See if the person needs CPR. If he does, give CPR. If you don't know how, give Hands-Only CPR.

Important

- Begin cooling the person immediately. Every minute counts.
- If you can't put the person in cool water up to her neck, cool her with a cool water spray.
- Stop cooling the person once her behavior is normal again. Continued cooling could lead to low body temperature (hypothermia).
- Only put water on the person's skin.
- If the person can drink, give her something to drink. Sports drinks are the best.
- If the person can't drink, wait for someone with more advanced training to arrive and take over.

What You Will Learn

In this section we'll cover

- Frostbite
- Low Body Temperature (Hypothermia)

Frostbite

Definitions and Key Facts

A cold injury to part of the body is called frostbite. Frostbite affects parts of the body that are exposed to the cold, such as the fingers, toes, nose, and ears. Frostbite typically occurs outside in cold weather. But it can also occur inside if workers don't have gloves on and handle cold materials, such as gases under pressure.

Signs

- The skin over the frostbitten area is white, waxy, or grayish-yellow.
- The frostbitten area is cold and numb.
- The frostbitten area is hard, and the skin doesn't move when you push it.

Actions for Frostbite

Step	Action
1	Move the person to a warm place.
2	Phone or ask someone to phone your emergency response number (or 911) and get the first aid kit.
3	Remove tight clothing and jewelry from the frostbitten part.
4	Remove wet clothing and pat the body dry. Put dry clothes on the person and cover the person with a blanket.
5	Do not try to thaw the frozen part if you think there may be a chance of refreezing.

Important

If you need to touch the frostbitten area, do so gently. Rubbing it may cause damage.

Low Body Temperature (Hypothermia)

Definitions and Key Facts

Hypothermia occurs when body temperature falls. Hypothermia is a serious condition that can cause death. A person can develop hypothermia even when the temperature is above freezing.

Shivering protects the body by producing heat. Shivering stops when the body becomes very cold.

Signs

- The skin is cool to the touch.
- Shivering (shivering stops when the body temperature is very low).
- The person may become confused or drowsy.
- Personality may change or the person may behave as if unconcerned about the condition.
- Muscles become stiff and rigid and the skin becomes ice cold and blue.

As the body temperature continues to drop

- The person stops responding
- The person's breathing slows
- It may be hard to tell whether the person is breathing
- The person may appear to be dead

Actions

Step	Action
1	Get the person out of the cold.
2	Remove wet clothing and pat the body dry. Put dry clothes on the person and cover the person with a blanket.
3	Phone or ask someone to phone your emergency response number (or 911) and get the first aid kit and AED, if available.
4	Wrap the person up with anything you have—clothing, towels, newspapers, etc. Cover the head but not the face.
5	See if the person needs CPR. If so, give CPR. If you don't know how, give Hands-Only CPR.

FYI: Rewarming

Place a person with low body temperature near a heat source and place containers of warm, but not hot, water in contact with the skin. It is important to get the person to medical care as soon as possible.

4. Poison Emergencies

What You Will Learn	In this section we'll cover the following: ■ Scene Safety for Poison Emergencies ■ Removing Poisons ■ Complete First Aid for Poison Emergencies

Definitions and Key Facts	A poison is anything someone swallows, breathes, or gets in the eyes or on the skin that causes sickness or death. Many products can poison people. This section will not deal with specific poisons. Instead it will cover general principles of first aid for a victim of poisoning. Follow your workplace guidelines about poisonous items in your workplace. The number for the American Association of Poison Control Centers (Poison Control) is 1-800-222-1222.

Scene Safety for Poison Emergencies

Definitions and Key Facts	If you think someone may have been exposed to a poison, make sure the scene is safe before giving first aid. This takes a few more steps than in other first aid situations.

Actions	

Step	Action
1	Make sure the scene is safe before you approach.
2	If the scene seems unsafe, do not approach. Tell everyone to move away.
3	Look for signs that warn you that poisons are nearby.
4	Look for spilled or leaking containers.
5	Stay out of the area with the poison if you see more than 1 victim.
6	If you approach the scene, wear appropriate protective equipment.

Removing Poisons

Definitions and Key Facts	Get the poison off the person as quickly as you safely can. Use lots of water to rinse the poisons off.

Actions

Step	Action
1	Make sure the scene is safe. Get the first aid kit. Wear PPE.
2	Help the person **take off contaminated clothing and jewelry**.
3	Quickly help the person to a **safety shower** or eyewash station if he responds and can move.
4	**Brush off** any dry powder or solid substances from the skin with your gloved hand.
5	**Rinse** the contaminated areas with a lot of water for at least 20 minutes or until someone with more training arrives and takes over.

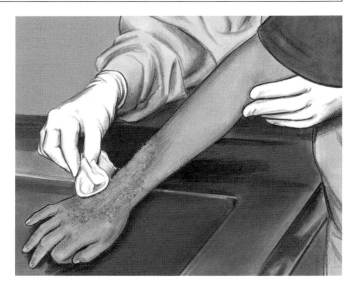

Figure 28. Brush off any dry powder or solid substances from the person's skin with your gloved hand.

Important

If only one eye is affected make sure the eye with the poison in it is the lower eye as you rinse. Make sure you do not rinse the poison into the unaffected eye.

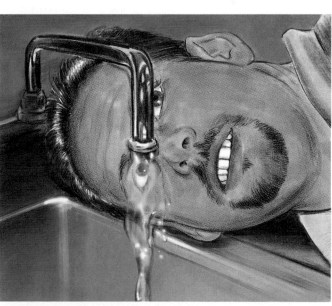

Figure 29. Help the person wash his eyes and face under water flowing from a faucet or hose. Or use an eyewash station.

Other First Aid for Poison Emergencies

Definitions and Key Facts

Worksites should have an MSDS (Material Safety Data Sheet) for each chemical at the worksite. You should know where the MSDS is at your worksite. The MSDS provides a description of how a specific poison can be harmful.

Unfortunately the MSDS usually provides little information about first aid actions. Some of the first aid actions listed in the MSDS or on the label of the poison may be outdated.

You will probably receive additional training on the MSDS during the "Right to Know" training your workplace provides.

Actions

Step	Action
1	Make sure the **scene is safe.** Get the first aid kit. Wear PPE.
2	Send someone to phone your **emergency response number (or 911).**
3	**Tell the dispatcher the name of the poison,** if possible.
4	**Remove the poison,** if possible.
5	Move the person from the scene of the poison if you can.
6	Help the person move to an area with fresh air, if possible.
7	Send someone to get the Material Safety Data Sheet (MSDS), if available.

Important

If you give CPR to a poisoning victim, use a mask for giving breaths if possible. This precaution is especially important if the poison is on the lips or mouth.

Some dispatchers may connect you to a poison control center. Give only those antidotes that the poison control center or dispatcher tells you to. The first aid instructions on the poison itself can be helpful but may be incomplete.

FYI

When you call the emergency response number, try to have the following information ready:

- What is the name of the poison? Can you describe it if you cannot name it?
- How much poison did the person touch, breathe, or swallow?
- About how old is the person? What is the person's approximate weight?
- When did the poisoning happen?
- How is the person feeling or acting now?

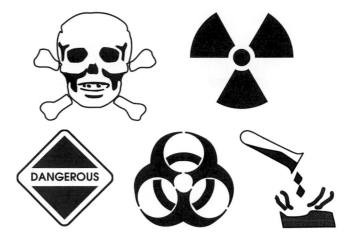

Figure 30. Look for symbols of poisons, such as these, nearby.

Review Questions: Environmental Emergencies

Question	Your Notes
1. Someone who has been bitten by an insect or bee may have a severe allergic reaction and should be watched for at least _____ minutes. a. 10 b. 20 c. 30 d. 60	
2. When someone has a bite be sure to wash the bite area with a lot of soap and water. True False	
3. Heat stroke is a life-threatening condition. True False	
4. Remove ticks _____. a. with a hot matchstick b. with lots of alcohol on the skin c. by using tweezers d. with your hands	

(continued)

Question	Your Notes
5. Being confused may be a symptom of heat stroke and low body temperature. True False	
6. If you give CPR to someone who has been poisoned it is important to use a mask, if possible, to give breaths. True False	

Answers: 1. c, 2. True, 3. True, 4. c, 5. True, 6. True

First Aid Skills Summary

Taking Off Gloves

- Grip 1 glove on the outside of the glove near the cuff and peel it down until it comes off inside out.
- Cup it with your other (gloved) hand.
- Place 2 fingers of your bare hand inside the cuff of the glove that is still on your hand.
- Peel that glove off so that it comes off inside out, with the first glove inside it.
- If there is blood on the gloves, dispose of the gloves properly.
- Put them in a biohazard waste bag or as required by your workplace.
- If you do not have a biohazard waste bag, put the gloves in a plastic bag that can be sealed before you dispose of it.
- Wash your hands after you give first aid so that you don't spread germs.

Finding the Problem

- Make sure the scene is safe and look for the cause of the problem.
- Tap and shout. If the person doesn't respond, phone your emergency response number (or 911) and get an AED. If the person responds, ask permission to help and ask what the problem is.
- Check breathing. If the person doesn't respond and isn't breathing or is only gasping, start CPR if you know how. If you don't know how, give Hands-Only CPR.
- Look for signs of injury, such as bleeding.
- Look for medical information jewelry.

Using Epinephrine Pens

- Get the prescribed epinephrine pen.
- Take off the safety cap. Follow the instructions on the pen.
- Hold the epinephrine pen in your fist without touching either end because the needle comes out of one end.
- Push the end with the needle hard against the side of the person's thigh, about halfway between the hip and knee. Give the injection through clothes or on bare skin.
- Hold the pen in place for about 10 seconds.
- Remove the needle and pen by pulling straight out.
- Rub the injection spot for about 10 seconds.
- After using the epinephrine pen, dispose of it properly.

- Note the time of the injection.
- Stay with the person until someone with more advanced training arrives and takes over.

How to Stop Bleeding You Can See

- Make sure the scene is safe. Get the first aid kit. Wear PPE.
- Place a dressing on the bleeding. Use the flat part of your fingers or the palm of your hand to apply pressure to the dressing.
- If the bleeding does not stop, add more dressings on top of the first and press harder.
- Keep pressure on the wound until it stops bleeding.
- If you can't keep pressure on the wound, wrap a bandage firmly over the dressings to hold them in place.

Bandaging

- Make sure the scene is safe. Get the first aid kit and wear PPE.
- Use direct pressure, with dressings if available, to stop any bleeding.
- Apply the bandage over the dressings.

Splinting Practice (Not Tested)

- Make sure the scene is safe. Get the first aid kit. Wear PPE.
- To make the splint, use something (such as a magazine) that will keep the arm or leg from moving, and pad the splint if possible.
- Ideally, place the splint so that it extends beyond the injured area and supports the joints above and below the injury.
- Tie the splint to the injured body part so that it supports the injured area. Use tape, gauze, or cloth to secure it.
- Make sure that the injured person is checked by a healthcare provider.

Part 5: CPR and AED

What You Will Learn

You'll learn when and how to provide CPR and use AEDs.

Topics Covered

- CPR and AED for Adults
- CPR and AED for Children
- How to Help a Choking Child
- CPR for Infants
- How to Help a Choking Infant

For information on adult choking, go to "Part 2: Medical Emergencies."

1. CPR and AED for Adults

What You Will Learn

In this section you'll learn when CPR is needed, how to give CPR to an adult, and how to use an AED.

Definitions and Key Facts

CPR stands for cardiopulmonary resuscitation. It consists of pushing on the chest (compressions) and giving breaths.

For the purpose of this course, an adult is anyone who has gone through or is going through puberty. When in doubt, treat someone as an adult.

Someone who "responds" moves, speaks, blinks, or otherwise reacts to you when you tap him and ask if he's OK. Someone who doesn't "respond" does nothing when you tap him and ask if he's OK.

Topics Covered

- Give CPR
- Use an AED
- Assess and Phone Your Emergency Response Number (or 911)
- Put It All Together

Give CPR: Compressions and Breaths

Definitions and Key Facts	CPR has 2 main parts: compressions and giving breaths.
	Pushing hard and fast on the chest is the most important part of CPR. When you push on the chest, you pump blood to the brain and heart.

Compressions

Definitions and Key Facts	A compression is the act of pushing on the chest.
	People often don't push hard enough because they're afraid of hurting the victim. An injury is unlikely, but it is better than death. It's better to push too hard than not hard enough.

Action: Push Hard and Push Fast

Follow these steps to push hard and push fast:

Step	Action
1	Make sure the person is lying on his back on a firm, flat surface.
2	Move clothes out of the way.
3	Put the heel of 1 hand on the lower half of the breastbone. Put the heel of your other hand on top of the first hand.
4	Push straight down **at least 2 inches** at a rate of **at least 100 compressions a minute.**
5	After each compression, let the **chest come back up** to its normal position.

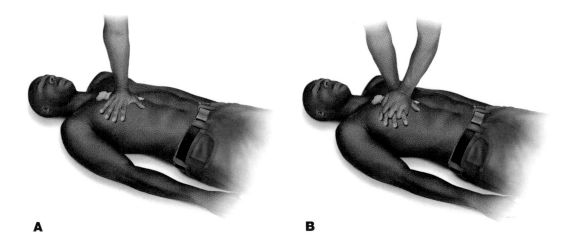

A   B

Figure 31. Compressions. **A,** Put the heel of 1 hand on the lower half of the breastbone. **B,** Put the other hand on top of the first hand.

FYI

Compressions are very important and doing them correctly is tiring. The more tired you are, the less effective your compressions are. If someone else knows CPR, take turns. Switch about every 2 minutes, moving quickly to keep the pause between compressions as short as possible. Remind each other to push down **at least 2 inches**, push at a rate of **at least 100 compressions a minute**, and let **the chest come back up** to its normal position after each compression.

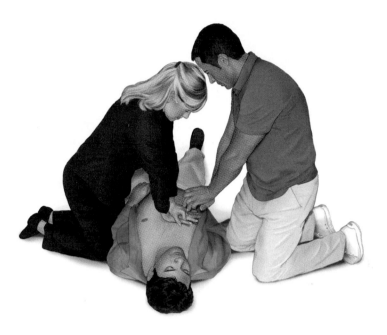

Figure 32. Switch rescuers.

Give Breaths

Definitions and Key Facts

Compressions are the most important part of CPR. If you're also able to give breaths, you will help even more. Your breaths need to make the chest rise. When the chest rises, you know the person has taken in enough air.

Action: Open the Airway

Before giving breaths, open the airway. Follow these steps to open the airway:

Step	Action
1	Put 1 hand on the forehead and the fingers of your other on the bony part of the chin.
2	Tilt the head back and lift the chin.

Important   Avoid pressing on the soft part of the neck or under the chin.

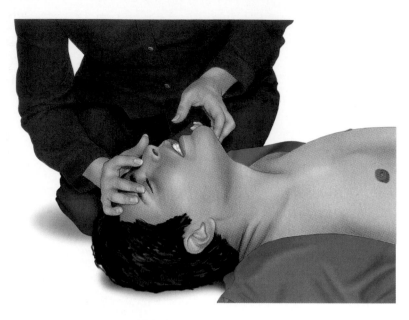

Figure 33. Open the airway with a head tilt–chin lift.

Actions: Give Breaths

Step	Action
1	While holding the airway open, pinch the nose closed.
2	Take a breath. Cover the person's mouth with your mouth.
3	Give 2 breaths (blow for 1 second each). Watch **for the chest to begin to rise** as you give each breath.

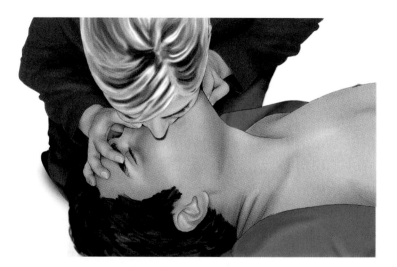

Figure 34. Give breaths.

Important

If you give someone a breath and the chest doesn't rise, allow the head to go back to its normal position. Then open the airway again by tilting the head and lifting the chin. Then give another breath. Make sure the chest rises.

Don't interrupt compressions for more than 10 seconds to give breaths. If the chest doesn't rise within 10 seconds, begin pushing hard and pushing fast on the chest again.

Using a Mask

Definitions and Key Facts

Giving breaths to another person is usually quite safe. During CPR there is very little chance that you will catch a disease. Even so, some workplaces require rescuers to have masks.

Masks are made of firm plastic and fit over the ill or injured person's mouth or mouth and nose. You may need to put the mask together before you use it.

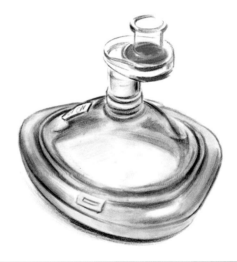

Figure 35. Some people use a mask when giving breaths.

Actions

Step	Action
1	Put the mask over the person's mouth and nose.
2	Tilt the head and lift the chin while pressing the mask against the person's face. It is important to make an airtight seal between the person's face and the mask while you lift the chin to keep the airway open.
3	Give 2 breaths (blow for 1 second each). Watch for the chest to begin to rise as you give each breath.

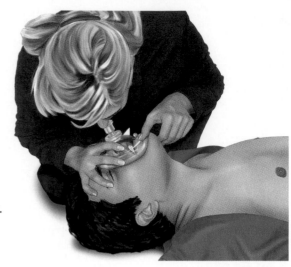

Figure 36. Giving breaths with a mask.

FYI

If the mask has a pointed end

- Put the narrow end of the mask at the top (bridge) of the nose
- Position the wide end so it covers the mouth.

Use an AED

Definitions and Key Facts

Sometimes a heart doesn't work right. An AED is a machine with a computer in it that can shock the heart and help it work properly again. If you start CPR right away and then use an AED within a few minutes, you will have the best chance of saving a life.

AEDs are safe, accurate, and easy to use. The AED will figure out if the person needs a shock and will tell you to give one if needed. It will even tell you when to make sure that no one is touching the person. The pads used to shock the person have a diagram showing you where to place them. Follow the diagram.

The most common ways to turn on an AED are to push an "ON" button or lift the lid of the AED. Once you turn on the AED, it will tell you everything you need to do.

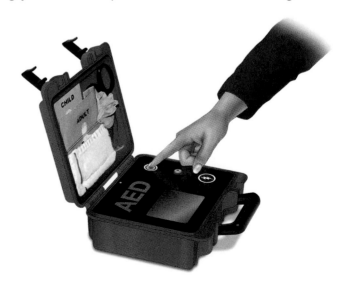

Figure 37. An AED.

Actions

Use an AED if someone doesn't respond and isn't breathing or is only gasping. There are 2 steps for using an AED:

Step	Action
1	Turn the AED on.
2	Follow the prompts you see and hear.

Important

If you have access to an AED, use it as quickly as possible. Make sure no one is touching the victim just before you push the "SHOCK" button. If you can't find an AED quickly, then start CPR. Push hard and push fast.

Figure 38. Make sure that no one is touching the person before giving a shock.

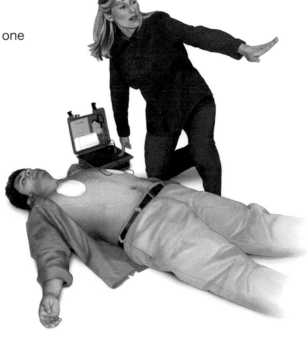

Figure 39. Placing pads on an adult.

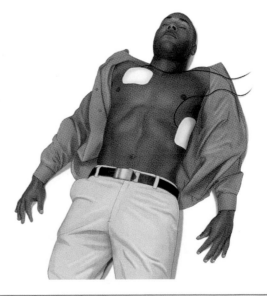

Assess and Phone Your Emergency Response Number (or 911)

Definitions and Key Facts	If a person doesn't respond and if that person isn't breathing or is only gasping, then you need to give CPR. If you are not sure whether to give CPR, go ahead and give it. It's better to give CPR to someone who doesn't need it than not to give it to someone who does need it.
Action: Make Sure the Scene Is Safe	Before you assess the need for CPR, make sure the scene is safe. Look for anything nearby that might hurt you. You don't want to hurt yourself.
Action: Tap and Shout	Check if the person responds. Tap him and shout, "Are you OK?" If he doesn't move, speak, blink, or otherwise react, then he is not responding.

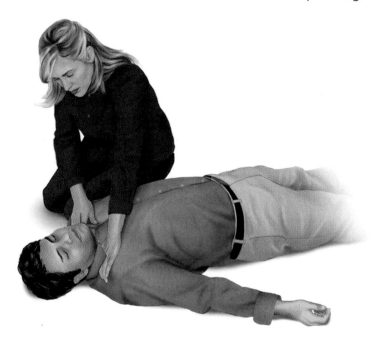

Figure 40. Tap and shout.

Action: Phone 911 and Get AED	If the person doesn't respond, it's important to get help. You or someone else (yell for help if you need to) should phone your emergency response number (or 911). Get an AED, if available.
Important	Stay on the phone until the 911 dispatcher (operator) tells you to hang up. Answering the dispatcher's questions will not delay the arrival of help.

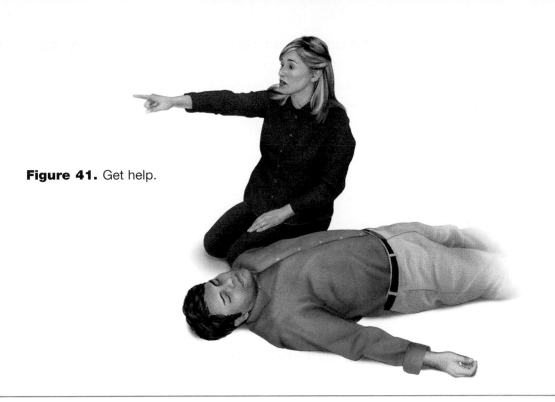

Figure 41. Get help.

**Action:
Check Breathing**

If the person doesn't respond, check his breathing. If the person isn't breathing at all or if he is only "gasping," then he needs CPR.

A person who gasps usually appears to be drawing air in very quickly. He may open his mouth and move the jaw, head, or neck. Gasps may appear forceful or weak, and some time may pass between gasps because they usually happen at a slow rate. The gasp may sound like a snort, snore, or groan. Gasping is not regular or normal breathing. It is a sign of cardiac arrest in someone who doesn't respond.

Figure 42. Check breathing.

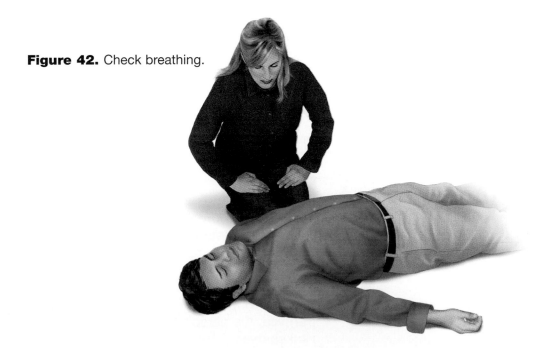

If the person is breathing but is not responding, roll him to his side and wait for someone with more advanced training to arrive and take over. Placing someone in the side position helps keep the airway clear in the event the person vomits. If the person stops breathing or is only gasping, you will need to roll him onto his back and assess the need for CPR.

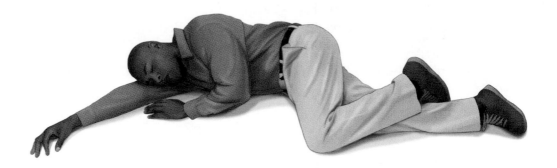

Figure 43. Side position.

Put It All Together

Definitions and Key Facts

When doing CPR, you **give sets of 30 compressions and 2 breaths**. Push straight down **at least 2 inches** at a rate of **at least 100 times a minute**. After each compression, let the **chest come back up** to its normal position.

Try not to interrupt compressions for more than 10 seconds, even when you give breaths.

Action: Adult CPR

Step	Action
1	Make sure the scene is safe.
2	Tap and shout.
3	Yell for help. You or someone else should phone the emergency response number (or 911) and get the AED.
4	Check breathing.
5	If the person isn't breathing or is only gasping, give CPR.
6	Give **30 compressions** at a **rate of at least 100 a minute** and a depth of **at least 2 inches.** After each compression, **let the chest come back up** to its normal position.
7	Open the airway and give **2 breaths.**
8	Keep giving sets of 30 compressions and 2 breaths until the AED arrives, the person starts to respond, or trained help arrives and takes over.

Adult CPR AED Skills Summary

Step	Action
1	**Make sure the scene is safe.**
2	**Tap and shout.** ■ Check to see if the person responds. ■ If the person doesn't respond, go to Step 3.
3	**Get help.** ■ Yell for help. ■ Have the person who comes phone 911 and get an AED. ■ If no one can help, phone 911 and get an AED. Use it.
4	**Check breathing.** ■ Make sure the person is on a firm, flat surface. ■ Check breathing. ■ If the person isn't breathing at all or is only gasping, give CPR. **No response** **+** **No breathing or only gasping** **=** **GIVE CPR**
5	**Push and give breaths. Give 30 compressions and 2 breaths.** ■ Compressions: – Move clothes out of the way. – Put the heel of 1 hand on the lower half of the breastbone. Put the heel of your other hand on top of the first hand. – Push straight down at least 2 inches at a rate of at least 100 compressions a minute. – After each compression, let the chest come back up to its normal position. – Compress the chest 30 times. ■ Breaths: – After 30 compressions, open the airway with a head tilt–chin lift. – After the airway is open, take a normal breath. – Pinch the nose shut. Cover the mouth with your mouth. – Give 2 breaths (blow for 1 second each). Watch for the chest to begin to rise as you give each breath. ■ AED: – Use it as soon as you have it. – Turn it on by lifting the lid or pressing the "ON" button. – Follow the prompts.
6	**Keep going.** ■ Keep giving sets of compressions and breaths until the person starts to breathe or move, or until someone with more advanced training arrives and takes over.

2. CPR and AED for Children

**What You
Will Learn**

In this section you'll learn when CPR is needed, how to give CPR to a child, and how to use an AED.

**Definitions and
Key Facts**

CPR is the act of pushing hard and pushing fast on the chest and giving breaths. CPR is given to someone whose heart has stopped pumping blood.

For purposes of this course, a child is someone who is older than 1 year and has not yet reached puberty. If you are in doubt about whether someone is an adult or child, treat as an adult.

A child who "responds" moves, speaks, blinks, or otherwise reacts to you when you tap him and ask if he's OK. A child who doesn't "respond" does nothing when you tap him and ask if he's OK.

Topics Covered

- Give CPR: Compressions and Breaths
- Use an AED
- Assess and Phone Your Emergency Response Number (or 911)
- Put It All Together

Give CPR: Compressions and Breaths

Compressions

**Definitions and
Key Facts**

Pushing hard and fast on the chest (compressions) is the most important part of CPR. When you push on the chest, you pump blood to the brain and heart.

People often don't push hard enough because they're afraid of hurting the child. An injury is unlikely, but it is better than death. It's better to push too hard than not hard enough.

**Action:
Push Hard and
Push Fast**

Follow these steps to push hard and push fast:

Step	Action
1	Make sure the child is lying on her back on a firm, flat surface.
2	Move clothes out of the way.
3	Put the heel of 1 hand on the lower half of the breastbone.
4	Push straight down **about 2 inches** at a rate of **at least 100 compressions a minute.**
5	After each compression, let the **chest come back up** to its normal position.

FYI

Use 1 hand for compressions. If you can't push down about 2 inches with 1 hand, use 2. One hand is not better than 2 or vice versa. Do what's necessary to push the chest down about 2 inches.

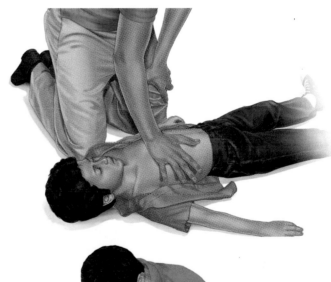

Figure 44. One-handed compressions.

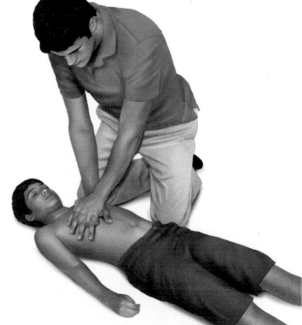

Figure 45. Two-handed compressions.

FYI

Compressions are important in CPR and doing them right is tiring. The more tired you are, the less effective your compressions are. If someone else knows CPR, take turns. Switch about every 2 minutes, moving quickly so that the pause in compressions is as short as possible. Remind each other to push down **about 2 inches,** to push at a rate of **at least 100 compressions a minute,** and to let the **chest come back up** to its normal position after each compression.

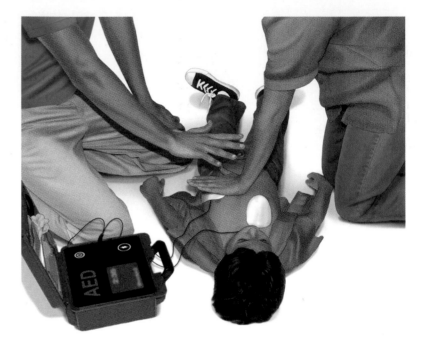

Figure 46. Switch rescuers.

Give Breaths

Definitions and Key Facts

Children often have healthy hearts. Usually, a child's heart stops because she can't breathe or is having trouble breathing. As a result, it's very important to give breaths as well as compressions to a child.

Your breaths need to make the child's chest rise. When the chest rises, you know the child has gotten enough air. Compressions are the most important part of CPR. If you are also able to give breaths, you will help the child even more.

Action: Open the Airway

Before giving breaths, open the airway. Follow these steps to open the airway:

Step	Action
1	Put 1 hand on the forehead and the fingers of your other on the bony part of the child's chin.
2	Tilt the head back and lift the chin.

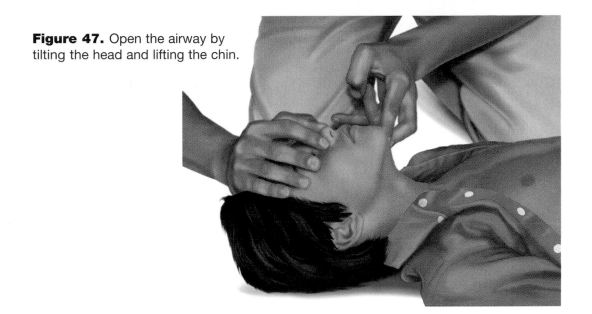

Figure 47. Open the airway by tilting the head and lifting the chin.

Important

Avoid pressing on the soft part of the neck or under the chin.

Action: Give Breaths

Follow these steps to give breaths to a child:

Step	Action
1	While holding the airway open, pinch the nose closed.
2	Take a breath. Cover the child's mouth with your mouth.
3	**Give 2 breaths** (blow for 1 second each). Watch for **the chest to begin to rise** as you give each breath.

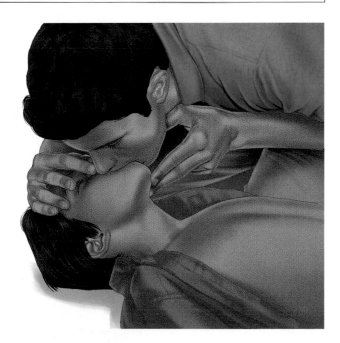

Figure 48. Cover the child's mouth with your mouth.

Important	If you give a child a breath and the chest doesn't rise, reopen the airway by allowing the head to go back to the normal position. Then open the airway again by tilting the head and lifting the chin. Then give another breath. Make sure the chest rises.
	Don't interrupt compressions for more than 10 seconds to give breaths. If the chest doesn't rise within 10 seconds, begin pushing hard and pushing fast on the chest again.

Using a Mask

Definitions and Key Facts	Giving breaths to another person is usually quite safe. During CPR there is very little chance that you will catch a disease. Even so, some workplaces require rescuers to have masks.
	Masks are made of firm plastic; they fit over the child's mouth or mouth and nose. You may need to put the mask together before you use it.

Actions

Step	Action
1	Put the mask over the child's mouth and nose.
2	Tilt the head and lift the chin while pressing the mask against the child's face. It is important to make an airtight seal between the child's face and the mask while you lift the chin to keep the airway open.
3	Give 2 breaths. Watch for the chest to begin to rise as you give each breath.

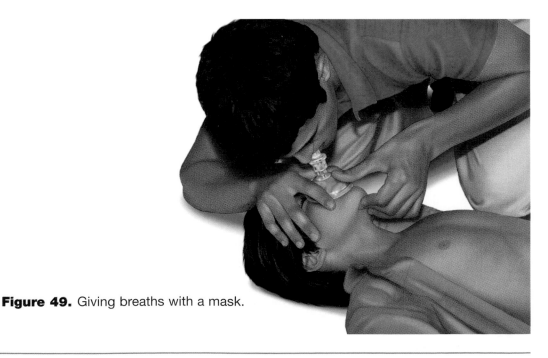

Figure 49. Giving breaths with a mask.

- Put the narrow end of the mask at the top (bridge) of the nose
- Position the wide end to cover the mouth

Use an AED

Definitions and Key Facts

If you start CPR right away and use an AED within a few minutes, you will have the best chance of saving a life.

AEDs are safe, accurate, and easy to use. The most common ways to turn on an AED are to push an "ON" button or lift the lid of the AED. Once you turn on the AED, it will tell you everything you need to do.

The AED will figure out if the child needs a shock and will tell you to give one if needed. It will even tell you when to make sure that no one is touching the child. The pads used to shock the child have a diagram showing you where to place them. Follow the diagram.

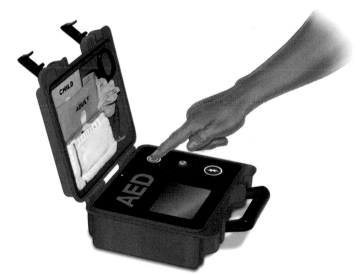

Figure 50. An automated external defibrillator (AED).

Action

Use an AED on any child who needs CPR. There are 4 simple steps for using an AED on a child:

Step	Action
1	Turn the AED on.
2	Look for child pads or for a child key or switch.
3	Use the child pads or turn the child key or switch.
4	Follow the prompts you see and hear.

Important	If there are no child pads or if there isn't a child key or switch, use the adult pads. Also, if the child is older than 8, use adult pads. (If you think the child might be 8 or older, assume he is, and use the adult pads.) When you put the pads on the chest, make sure they don't touch each other. If a child is very small, you may need to put 1 pad on the child's chest and the other on the child's back.
	If you have access to an AED, use it as quickly as possible. Make sure no one is touching the child just before pushing the "SHOCK" button. If you can't find an AED quickly, don't wait. Start CPR.

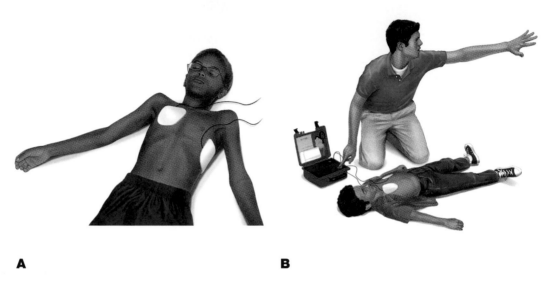

A   **B**

Figure 51. A, Placing child pads on a child. **B,** Making sure no one is touching the child.

Assess and Phone Your Emergency Response Number (or 911)

Definitions and Key Facts	Now that you've learned how to give CPR, it's time to learn when to give CPR. If a child doesn't respond and if that child isn't breathing or is only gasping, then you need to give CPR.
	If you are not sure whether to give CPR, go ahead and give it. It's better to give CPR to someone who doesn't need it than not to give it to someone who does need it.
Action: Make Sure the Scene Is Safe	Before you give CPR, make sure the scene is safe. Look for anything nearby that might hurt you. You don't want to hurt yourself.

**Action:
Tap and Shout**

Check if the child responds. Tap him and shout, "Are you OK?" If he doesn't move, speak, blink, or otherwise react, then he is not responding.

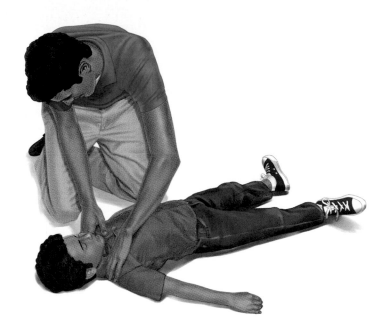

Figure 52. Tap and shout.

**Action:
Yell for Help**

Yell for help. If someone comes, have that person phone 911 and get an AED. Whether or not someone comes, check the child's breathing next.

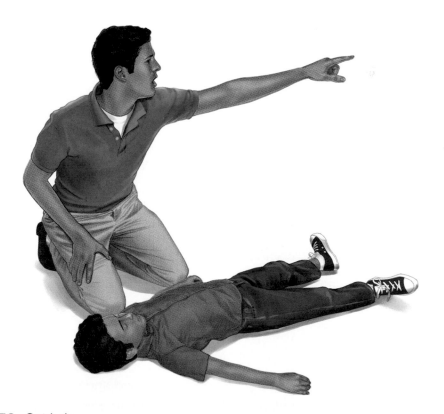

Figure 53. Get help.

Action:
Check Breathing

If the child doesn't respond, check his breathing. If the child isn't breathing at all or if he is only "gasping," then he needs CPR.

A person who gasps usually appears to be drawing air in very quickly. He may open his mouth and move the jaw, head, or neck. Gasps may appear forceful or weak, and some time may pass between gasps as they usually happen at a slow rate. The gasp may sound like a snort, snore, or groan. Gasping is not regular or normal breathing. It is a sign of cardiac arrest in someone who doesn't respond.

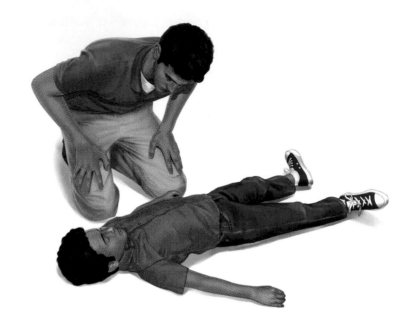

Figure 54. Check breathing.

Put It All Together

Definitions and Key Facts

Since children's hearts are often healthy and since breathing trouble is often the cause of the child's heart problem, it's important to get air to the child as fast as possible. For this reason, you should give 5 sets of CPR before phoning for help or getting an AED. (If someone else is nearby, send that person to phone for help and get an AED as quickly as possible.)

Compressions are very important; they are the core of CPR. Try not to interrupt compressions for more than a few seconds, even when you give breaths.

Action:
Give 5 Sets of CPR

When doing CPR, you **give sets of 30 compressions and 2 breaths.** Push down **about 2 inches** at a rate of at **least 100 times a minute.** After each push, let the **chest come back up** to its normal position.

If the child doesn't respond and isn't breathing or is only gasping, give him 5 sets of CPR (1 set = 30 compressions and 2 breaths).

| Action:
**Phone and Get
an AED** | After 5 sets of CPR, phone 911 and get an AED, if no one has done this yet. As soon as you have the AED, use it. |

| Action:
Keep Going | After phoning 911, keep giving sets of 30 compressions and 2 breaths until the child begins to respond or until someone with more advanced training arrives and takes over. |

| **FYI:
Answering
Dispatcher
Questions** | You need to stay on the phone until the 911 dispatcher (operator) tells you to hang up. |

The dispatcher will ask you about the emergency. She may also tell you how to help the child until someone with more advanced training arrives and takes over.

Answering the dispatcher's questions will not delay the arrival of help. If you can, take the phone with you so that you are beside the child while you talk to the dispatcher.

**Action:
Child CPR**

No breathing

No response + **or** = **GIVE CPR**

only gasping

The following table shows the steps for child CPR:

Step	Action
1	Make sure the scene is safe.
2	Tap and shout.
3	Yell for help.
4	Check breathing.
5	If the child isn't responding and either isn't breathing or is only gasping, **give 5 sets of 30 compressions and 2 breaths; then phone 911 and get an AED.**
6	Keep giving **sets of compressions and breaths** until the child starts to speak, breathe, or move, or until someone with more advanced training arrives and takes over.

Important

If another person is with you when you give CPR—or if you can yell for help and get someone to come help you—then send the other person to phone 911 while you start pushing hard and fast and giving breaths. **You give compressions and breaths; the other person phones and gets the AED.**

The following table summarizes differences between adult and child CPR:

What's Different	What to Do for an Adult	What to Do for a Child
When to phone the emergency response number or 911	Phone after checking for a response.	Phone after giving 5 sets of compressions and breaths if you are alone.
Using an AED	Use the adult pads.	• Look for a child key or switch. • Use the child pads. • If there are no child pads, use the adult pads. • If you use adult pads, make sure the pads don't touch each other.
Compression depth	Push down at least 2 inches.	Push down about 2 inches.

Child CPR AED Skills Summary

Step	Action
1	**Make sure the scene is safe.**
2	**Tap and shout.** ■ Check to see if the person responds. ■ If the person doesn't respond, go to Step 3.
3	**Yell for help.** ■ See if someone can help you. ■ Have that person phone 911 and get an AED.
4	**Check breathing.** ■ Make sure the child is on a firm flat surface. ■ See if the child is not breathing at all or only gasping. No response + **No breathing or only gasping** = **GIVE CPR**

5	**Give CPR. Give 5 sets of 30 compressions and 2 breaths, and then phone 911 and get an AED (if no one has done this yet).**
	■ Compressions:
	  – Move clothes out of the way.
	  – Put the heel of 1 hand on the lower half of the breastbone.
	  – Push straight down about 2 inches at a rate of at least 100 compressions a minute.
	  – After each compression, let the chest come back up to its normal position.
	  – Compress the chest 30 times.
	■ Breaths:
	  – After 30 compressions, open the airway with a head tilt–chin lift.
	  – After the airway is open, take a normal breath.
	  – Pinch the nose shut. Cover the child's mouth with your mouth.
	  – Give 2 breaths (blow for 1 second each). Watch for the chest to begin to rise as you give each breath.
	■ AED:
	  – Use it as soon as you have it.
	  – Turn it on by lifting the lid or pressing the "ON" button.
	  – Use child pads or child key or switch. (Use adult pads if no child pads are available.)
	  – Follow the prompts.

6	**Keep going.** ■ Keep giving sets of compressions and breaths until the child starts to breathe or move, or until someone with more advanced training arrives and takes over.

3. How to Help a Choking Child

**What You
Will Learn**

In this section you'll learn the signs of choking and how to help a choking child.

**Definitions and
Key Facts**

Choking is when food or another object gets stuck in the airway or throat. The object stops air from getting to the lungs.

Some choking is mild and some is severe. If it's severe, act fast. Get the object out so the child can breathe.

Topics

- Mild vs Severe Choking
- How to Help a Choking Child
- How to Help a Choking Child Who Stops Responding

Mild vs Severe Choking

Action

Use the following table to figure out if a child has mild or severe choking and what you should do:

If the child	The block in the airway is	And you should
• Can make sounds • Can cough loudly	Mild	• Stand by and let her cough • If you are worried about her breathing, phone your emergency response number (or 911)
• Cannot breathe or • Has a cough that has no sound or • Cannot talk or make a sound or • Makes the choking sign	Severe	• Act quickly • Follow the steps to help a choking child

**FYI:
The Choking Sign**

A child who is choking might use the choking sign (holding the neck with one or both hands).

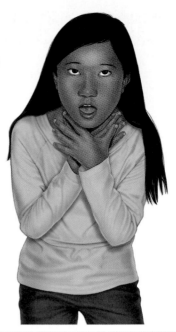

Figure 55. The choking sign: holding the neck with one or both hands.

How to Help a Choking Child

Definitions and Key Facts

When a child has severe choking, give thrusts slightly above the belly button. These thrusts are sometimes called the Heimlich maneuver. Like a cough, each thrust pushes air from the lungs. This can help remove an object that is blocking the airway.

Action: Help a Choking Child

Follow these steps to help a choking child:

Step	Action
1	If you think the child is choking, ask, "Are you choking?" If he nods yes, tell him you are going to help.
2	**Get behind him.** Wrap your arms around him so that your hands are in front.
3	**Make a fist** with 1 hand.
4	Put the thumb side of your fist slightly above the belly button and well below the breastbone.
5	**Grasp the fist with your other hand** and give quick upward thrusts into the abdomen.
6	**Give thrusts** until the object is forced out and he can breathe, cough, or talk, or until he stops responding.

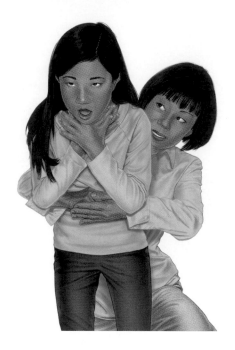

Figure 56. Helping a choking child.

Action: Help a Choking Large Child

If the choking child is very large and you can't wrap your arms fully around the waist, give thrusts on the chest instead of thrusts on the abdomen.

Follow the same steps except for the location where you place your arms and hands. Put your arms under the child's armpits and your hands on the lower half of the breastbone. Pull straight back to give the chest thrusts.

Figure 57. Chest thrusts on a choking large child.

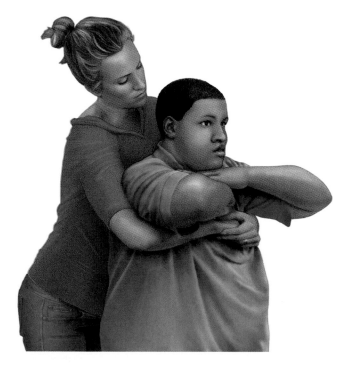

FYI

A child who has been given thrusts should see a healthcare provider.

Definitions and Key Facts

If you give a child thrusts but you can't remove the object blocking the airway, the child will stop responding. Pushing on his chest may force the object out.

Action: Help a Child Who Stops Responding

If the child stops responding, follow these steps:

Step	Action
1	Lower the child to a firm flat surface.
2	Tap and shout.
3	**Yell for help.**
4	**Check breathing.**
5	**Give 30 compressions.**
6	After 30 compressions, open the airway. **If you see an object in the mouth, take it out.**
7	**Give 2 breaths.**
8	**Repeat** giving **sets of 30 compressions and 2 breaths**, checking the mouth for objects after each set of compressions.
9	**After 5 sets of 30 compressions and 2 breaths, phone** your emergency response number (or 911) and get an AED.
10	**Give sets of 30 compressions and 2 breaths**, checking the mouth for objects after each set of compressions until the child starts to respond or until someone with more advanced training arrives and takes over.

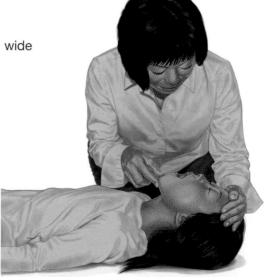

Figure 58. Open the child's mouth wide and look for the object.

Important	If another person is with you when the child stops responding—or if you can yell for help and get someone to come help you—send the other person to phone the emergency response number or (911) and get an AED while you start pushing hard and fast and giving breaths. **You give compressions and breaths; the other person phones and gets the AED.**

4. CPR for Infants

What You Will Learn	In this section you'll learn when to give CPR and how to give CPR to an infant.

Definitions and Key Facts	CPR is the act of pushing hard and pushing fast on the chest and giving breaths. CPR is given to someone whose heart has stopped pumping blood.
	For purposes of this course, an infant is someone who is younger than 1 year.
	An infant who "responds" moves, makes sounds, blinks, or otherwise reacts to you when you tap him and shout his name. An infant who doesn't "respond" does nothing when you tap him and shout.

Topics Covered	■ Give CPR
	■ Assess and Phone Your Emergency Response Number (or 911)
	■ Put It All Together

Give CPR: Compressions and Breaths

Compressions

Definitions and Key Facts	Pushing hard and fast on the chest (compressions) is the most important part of CPR. When you push on the chest, you pump blood to the brain and heart.
	People often don't push hard enough because they're afraid of hurting the infant. An injury is unlikely, but it is better than death. It's better to push too hard than not hard enough.
	If possible, place the infant on a firm, flat surface above the ground, such as a table. This makes it easier to give CPR.

Action: Push Hard and Push Fast

Follow these steps to push hard and push fast:

Step	Action
1	Make sure the infant is lying on her back on a firm, flat surface. If possible, use a surface above the ground.
2	Move clothes out of the way.
3	Put 2 fingers of 1 hand on the breastbone just below the nipple line.
4	Press the infant's chest straight down about **1½ inches** at a rate of **at least 100 compressions a minute.**
5	After each compression, let the **chest come back up** to its normal position.

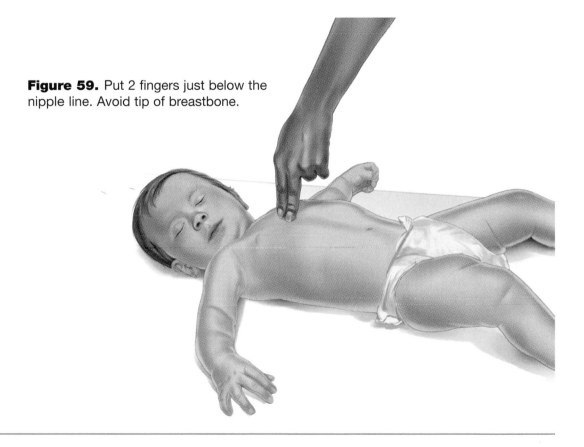

Figure 59. Put 2 fingers just below the nipple line. Avoid tip of breastbone.

FYI

Compressions are important in CPR and doing them correctly is tiring. The more tired you are, the less effective your compressions are. If someone else knows CPR, take turns. Switch about every 2 minutes, moving quickly so that the pause in compressions is as short as possible. Remind each other to push down about **1½ inches**, to push at a rate of **at least 100 compressions a minute,** and to let the **chest come back up** to its normal position after each compression.

Give Breaths

Definitions and Key Facts

Infants often have healthy hearts. Usually, an infant's heart stops because she can't breathe or is having trouble breathing. As a result, it's very important to give breaths as well as compressions to an infant.

Your breaths need to make the infant's chest rise. When the chest rises, you know the infant has gotten enough air. Compressions are the most important part of CPR. If you are also able to give breaths, you will help the infant even more.

Action: Open the Airway

Before giving breaths, open the airway. Follow these steps to open the airway:

Step	Action
1	Put 1 hand on the forehead and the fingers of your other on the bony part of the infant's chin.
2	Tilt the head back and lift the chin.

Important

When tilting an infant's head, do not push it back too far because this may block the infant's airway. Avoid pressing the soft part of the neck or under the chin.

**Action:
Give Breaths**

Follow these steps to give breaths to an infant:

Step	Action
1	While holding the infant's airway open, take a normal breath.
2	Cover the infant's mouth and nose with your mouth.
3	**Give 2 breaths** (blow for 1 second each). Watch for **the chest to begin to rise** as you give each breath.

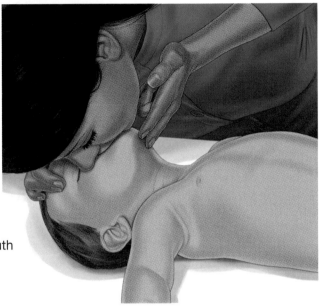

Figure 60. Cover the infant's mouth and nose with your mouth.

**FYI:
Tips for Giving Breaths**

If your mouth is too small to cover the infant's mouth and nose, put your mouth over the infant's nose and give breaths through the infant's nose. (You may need to hold the infant's mouth closed to stop air from coming out through the mouth.)

Important

If you give an infant a breath and the chest doesn't rise, reopen the airway by allowing the head to go back to the normal position. Then open the airway again by tilting the head and lifting the chin. Then give another breath. Make sure the chest rises.

Don't interrupt compressions for more than 10 seconds to give breaths. If the chest doesn't rise within 10 seconds, begin pushing hard and pushing fast on the chest again.

Definitions and Key Facts

Giving breaths to another person is usually quite safe. During CPR there is very little chance that you will catch a disease. Even so, some workplaces require rescuers to have masks.

Masks are made of firm plastic and fit over the infant's mouth or mouth and nose. You may need to put the mask together before you use it.

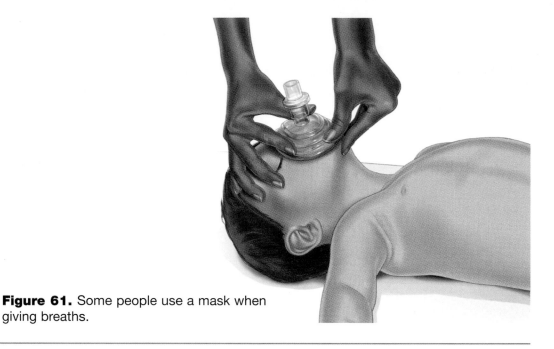

Figure 61. Some people use a mask when giving breaths.

Actions

Step	Action
1	Put the mask over the infant's mouth and nose.
2	Tilt the head and lift the chin while pressing the mask against the infant's face. It is important to make an airtight seal between the infant's face and the mask while you lift the chin to keep the airway open.
3	Give 2 breaths. Watch for the chest to begin to rise as you give each breath.

FYI

If the mask has a pointed end

- Put the narrow end of the mask at the top (bridge) of the nose
- The wide end should cover the mouth.

Assess and Phone Your Emergency Response Number (or 911)

Definitions and Key Facts

Now that you've learned how to give CPR, it's time to learn when to give CPR. If an infant doesn't respond and if that infant isn't breathing or is only gasping, you need to give CPR.

If you are not sure whether to give CPR, go ahead and give it. It's better to give CPR to someone who doesn't need it than not to give it to someone who does need it.

Action:
Make Sure the Scene Is Safe

Before you give CPR, make sure the scene is safe. Look for anything nearby that might hurt you. You don't want to hurt yourself.

Action:
Tap and Shout

Check if the infant responds. Tap his foot and shout his name. If he doesn't move, make a sound, blink, or otherwise react, he is not responding.

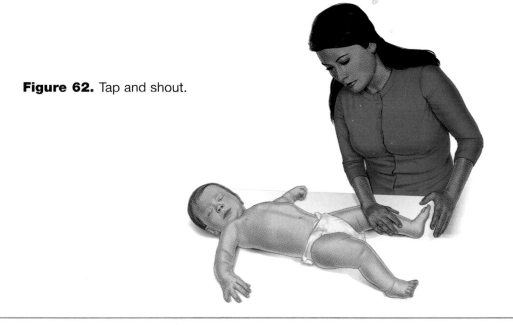

Figure 62. Tap and shout.

Action:
Yell for Help

Yell for help. If someone comes, have that person phone 911. Whether someone comes or not, check the infant's breathing next.

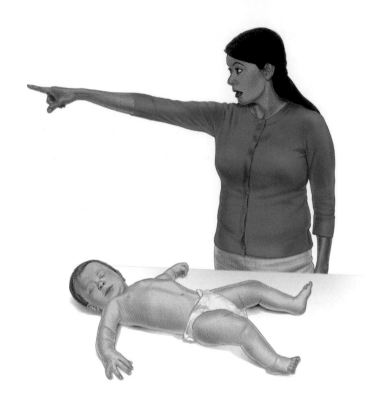

Figure 63. Get help.

**Action:
Check Breathing**

If the infant doesn't respond, check his breathing. If the infant isn't breathing at all or if he is only "gasping," then he needs CPR.

A person who gasps usually appears to be drawing air in very quickly. He may open his mouth and move his jaw, head, or neck. Gasps may appear forceful or weak, and some time may pass between gasps as they usually happen at a slow rate. The gasp may sound like a snort, snore, or groan. Gasping is not regular or normal breathing. It is a sign of cardiac arrest in someone who doesn't respond.

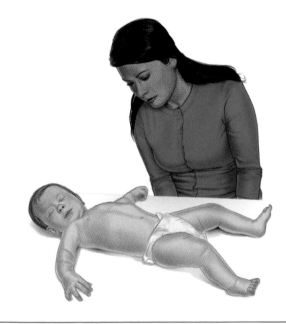

Figure 64. Check breathing.

Put It All Together

Definitions and Key Facts

Since infants' hearts are often healthy and since breathing trouble is often the cause of the infant's heart problem, it's important to get air to the infant as quickly as possible. For this reason, you should give 5 cycles of CPR before phoning for help. (If someone else is nearby, send that person to phone for help as soon as possible.)

Compressions are very important and are the core of CPR. Try not to interrupt compressions for more than a few seconds, even when you give breaths.

Action: Give 5 Sets of CPR

When doing CPR on an infant, **give sets of 30 compressions and 2 breaths.** Push down about **1½ inches** at a rate of at **least 100 times a minute.** After each push, let the **chest come back up** to its normal position.

If the infant is not injured and you are alone, after 5 sets of 30 compressions and 2 breaths, you may carry the infant with you to phone 911.

Figure 65. Phone your emergency response number (or 911).

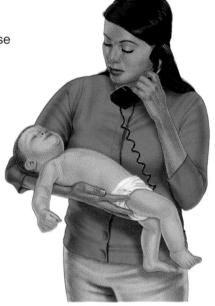

Action: Phone 911

After 5 sets of CPR, phone 911 if no one has done this yet. Take the infant with you to the phone if possible.

Action: Keep Going

After phoning, keep giving sets of 30 compressions and 2 breaths until the infant begins to respond or until someone with more advanced training arrives and takes over.

You need to stay on the phone until the 911 dispatcher (operator) tells you to hang up.

The dispatcher will ask you about the emergency. She may also tell you how to help the infant until someone with more advanced training arrives and takes over.

Answering the dispatcher's questions will not delay the arrival of help. If you can, take the phone with you or carry the infant with you so that you're with the infant while you talk to the dispatcher.

**Action:
Infant CPR**

| No response | + | No breathing or only gasping | = | GIVE CPR |

The following table shows the steps for infant CPR:

Step	Action
1	Make sure the scene is safe.
2	Tap and shout.
3	Yell for help.
4	Check breathing.
5	If the infant isn't responding and either isn't breathing or is only gasping, **give 5 sets of 30 compressions and 2 breaths, and then phone 911.**
6	Keep giving **sets of compressions and breaths** until the infant starts to breathe or move, or until someone with more advanced training arrives and takes over.

Important

If another person is with you when you give CPR—or if you can yell for help and get someone to come help you—then send the other person to phone 911 while you start pushing hard and fast and giving breaths. **You give compressions and breaths; the other person phones.**

Infant CPR Skills Summary

Step	Action
1	**Make sure the scene is safe.**
2	**Tap and shout.** ■ Check to see if the infant responds. ■ If the infant doesn't respond, go to Step 3.
3	**Yell for help.** ■ See if someone can help you. ■ Have that person phone 911.
4	**Check breathing.** ■ Make sure the infant is on a firm flat surface. If possible, use a surface above the ground. ■ See if the infant isn't breathing or is only gasping. **No response** + **No breathing or only gasping** = **GIVE CPR**
5	**Give CPR. Give 5 sets of 30 compressions and 2 breaths, and then phone 911 (if no one has phoned yet).** ■ Compressions: – Move clothes out of the way. – Place 2 fingers just below the nipple line. – Push straight down about 1½ inches at a rate of at least 100 compressions a minute. – After each compression, let the chest come back up to its normal position. ■ Breaths: – After 30 compressions, open the airway with a head tilt–chin lift. – After the airway is open, take a normal breath. – Cover the infant's mouth and nose with your mouth. – Give 2 breaths (blow for 1 second each). Watch for the chest to begin to rise as you give each breath.
6	**Keep going.** ■ Keep giving sets of 30 compressions and 2 breaths until the infant starts to breathe or move, or until someone with more advanced training arrives and takes over.

5. How to Help a Choking Infant

What You Will Learn

In this section you'll learn the signs of choking in an infant and how to help a choking infant.

Definitions

Choking is when food or another object gets stuck in the airway or throat. The object stops air from getting to the lungs.

Some choking is mild and some is severe. If it's severe, act fast. Get the object out so the infant can breathe.

Topics

- Mild vs Severe Choking
- How to Help a Choking Infant
- How to Help a Choking Infant Who Stops Responding

Mild vs Severe Choking

Action

Use the following table to figure out if an infant has mild or severe choking and what you should do.

If the infant	The block in the airway is	And you should
• Can make sounds • Can cough loudly	Mild	• Stand by and let her cough • If you are worried about the infant's breathing, phone 911
• Cannot breathe or • Has a cough that has no sound or • Cannot make a sound	Severe	• Act quickly • Follow the steps to help a choking infant

How to Help a Choking Infant

Definitions and Key Facts

When an infant has severe choking, use back slaps and chest thrusts to help remove the object blocking the airway.

**Action:
Help a Choking
Infant**

Step	Action
1	Hold the infant facedown on your forearm. Support the infant's head and jaw with your hand.
2	Give up to **5 back slaps** with the heel of your other hand between the infant's shoulder blades.
3	If the object does not come out after 5 back slaps, turn the infant onto his back, supporting the head.
4	Give up to **5 chest thrusts** using 2 fingers of your other hand to push on the chest in the same place you push during CPR.
5	**Repeat** giving 5 back slaps and 5 chest thrusts until the infant can breathe, cough, or cry or until he stops responding.

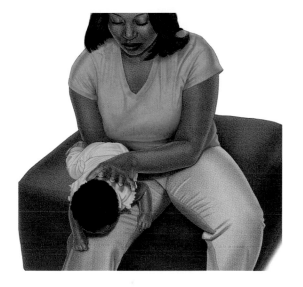

Figure 66. Give up to 5 back slaps.

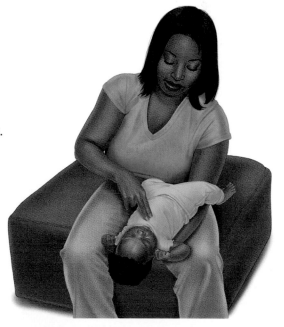

Figure 67. Give up to 5 chest thrusts.

An infant who has been given back slaps and chest thrusts should be seen by a healthcare provider.

How to Help a Choking Infant Who Stops Responding

Definitions and Key Facts

If you give an infant back slaps and chest thrusts and can't remove the object blocking the airway, the infant will stop responding. Pushing on his chest may force the object out.

Action: Help a Choking Infant Who Stops Responding

If the infant stops responding, follow these steps:

Step	Action
1	Place the infant faceup on a firm, flat surface above the ground, such as a table.
2	Tap and shout.
3	**Yell for help.**
4	**Check breathing.**
5	**Compress the chest 30 times.**
6	After 30 compressions, open the airway. **If you see an object in the mouth, take it out.**
7	**Give 2 breaths.**
8	**Repeat** giving **sets of 30 compressions and 2 breaths,** checking the mouth for objects after each set of compressions.
9	**After 5 sets of 30 compressions and 2 breaths, phone your emergency response number (or 911).**
10	**Give sets of 30 compressions and 2 breaths,** checking the mouth for objects after each set of compressions until the infant starts to respond or until someone with more advanced training arrives and takes over.

Important

Give only back slaps and chest thrusts to an infant. Giving thrusts to his abdomen could cause serious harm.

If another person is with you when the infant stops responding—or if you can yell for help and get someone to come help you—send the other person to phone the emergency response number (or 911) while you start pushing hard and fast and giving breaths. **You give compressions and breaths; the other person phones.**

Conclusion

Congratulations on completing this course.

Practice your skills often. This will keep them fresh and help you prepare for an emergency. It's important to phone the emergency response number (or 911) when an emergency arises. The operator also may be able to remind you what to do.

Contact the American Heart Association if you want more information on CPR, AEDs, or first aid. You can visit **www.heart.org/cpr** or call 1-877-AHA-4CPR (877-242-4277) to find a class near you.

Even if you don't remember all the steps exactly, it is important for you to try. Any help, even if it isn't perfect, is better than no help at all.

Summary of CPR and AED for Adults, Children, and Infants

Action	Adult and Older Child (has gone through or is going through puberty)	Child (1 to puberty)	Infant (less than 1 year old)
Check for response	Tap and shout		
Phone your emergency response number (or 911)	Phone your emergency response number (or 911) as soon as you find that the person does not respond	Phone your emergency response number (or 911) after giving 5 sets of 30 compressions and 2 breaths (if you are alone)	
• Give compressions			
• Compression location	Lower half of the breastbone		Just below the nipple line
• Compression method	2 hands	1 or 2 hands	2 fingers
• Compression depth	At least 2 inches	About 2 inches	About 1½ inches
• Compression rate	At least 100 a minute		
• Sets of compressions and breaths	30:2		
Open the airway Use a head tilt–chin lift	Head tilt–chin lift		Head tilt–chin lift (do not tilt the head back too far)
Check breathing	Look for only gasping or no breathing (take at least 5 seconds but no more than 10 seconds)		
Start CPR	Give sets of 30 compressions and 2 breaths (1 second each)		
AED • Press the "ON" button or open the lid	Use the AED as soon as it arrives		
• Attach pads to the person's bare chest	Use adult pads	Use child pads/key/switch if child is between 1 and 8 years old or adult pads if child is 8 or older	
• Follow the AED prompts			

Index